Proceedings in Life Sciences

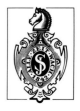

Molecular Aspects of Neurobiology

Edited by
Rita Levi Montalcini, Pietro Calissano,
Eric R. Kandel, and Adriana Maggi

With 73 Figures

Springer-Verlag
Berlin Heidelberg New York Tokyo

Prof. Dr. Rita Levi Montalcini
Dr. Pietro Calissano
Institute of Cell Biology, CNR
Via Romagnosi 18/A
I-00196 Rome, Italy

Dr. Eric Richard Kandel
Center for Neurobiology and Behavior
Columbia University
College of Physicians and Surgeons
722 West 168th Street
New York, NY 10032, USA

Dr. Adriana Maggi
Institute of Pharmacology and Pharmacognosy
University of Milano
Piazza Durante 11
I-20131 Milano, Italy

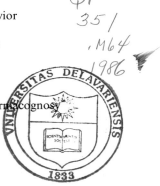

Cover illustration:
Rat superior cervical ganglia cells cultivated in presence of NGF.
Photograph Luigi Aloe.

ISBN 3-540-15776-X Springer-Verlag Berlin Heidelberg New York Tokyo
ISBN 0-387-15776-X Springer-Verlag New York Heidelberg Berlin Tokyo

Library of Congress Cataloging in Publication Data. Molecular aspects of neurobiology. (Proceedings in life sciences). Includes bibliographies and index. 1. Neurophysiology – Congresses. 2. Molecular biology – Congresses. 3. Neurogenetics – Congresses. I. Levi Montalcini, Rita. II. Series. [DNLM: 1. Neurobiology. 2. Neurophysiology. WL 102 M7183]. QP351.M64 1986 599.188 86-10215.

Printing and bookbinding: Brühlsche Universitätsdruckerei, Giessen
2131/3130-543210

Preface

The past two decades may well become known as the golden era of neurobiology. This field, that in the first half of this century seemed far too complex to be investigated with the low resolution techniques available to the investigators, suddenly blossomed in the second half of the century into one of the most promising areas of biology, thanks to discoveries which took place practically simultaneously in most areas of neurobiological research.

Here we mention only some of the most important: the discovery of the large number of neurotransmitters from monoamines to peptides, the identification of the mechanism of action of different agents through their binding to specific receptors, the recognition that neurotransmitters act most of the time through a second messenger, and the discovery that growth and differentiation of nerve cells depend on activation by the protein molecule; all these were recognized as specific growth facts, of which the NGF was both the first to be discovered and the object of the most intensive investigation.

Recently, the development of highly sophisticated techniques such as recombinant DNA and monoclonal antibodies has been successfully applied at the cellular and subcellular level to the study of nerve cells, neuronal cell population, and to the mechanism of their interaction.

Studies pursued with the collaboration of different investigators all over the world have opened a new panorama of the tremendous complexity of the CNS, from the neuron to the whole organism.

It was the object of the conference held in Florence in June 1985 under the sponsorship of Fondazione Lorenzini to bring together experts in different areas of neurobiology. This volume, a selection of the papers presented at the Symposium *Molecular Aspects of Neurobiology*, provides a picture of the state of the art and of the perspectives opened by these new powerful approaches to the study of the structure and function of the nervous system.

Rita Levi Montalcini
Rodolfo Paoletti

Contents

Contributors

You will find the addresses at the beginning of the respective contributions

Interrelationships of Cellular Mechanisms for Different Forms of Learning and Memory

P. MONTAROLO, S. SCHACHER, V.F. CASTELLUCCI, R.D. HAWKINS, T.W. ABRAMS, P. GOELET, and E.R. KANDEL[1]

1. Introduction

The recent increase in technical and conceptual strength of both psychology and biology makes it possible to begin to examine problems at the boundary between the two disciplines. One particularly important set of problems at this boundary concerns the study of learning and memory. *Learning* refers to the acquisition of new knowledge about the environment and *memory* refers to the retention of that knowledge. Learning and memory are universal features of nervous systems. All animals possess the capability for elementary forms of learning and several forms of learning first described in mammals, such as habituation, sensitization, classical conditioning, and operant conditioning, have been shown to be formally similar throughout phylogeny. This observation has encouraged the use of higher invertebrates, which offer the advantage of particularly simple nervous systems in which various forms of learning can be studied effectively on the cellular level.

In turn, the study of learning in animals with simple nervous systems has two goals. The first goal is to use this simplicity to analyze the molecular mechanisms underlying learning and memory. A second, less obvious but equally important goal is to use cell and molecular approaches to gain insights into the mechanistic interrelationship between various forms of learning. How does long-term memory relate to short-term memory? Do nonassociative forms of learning use similar or different cellular mechanisms than associative forms of learning?

In this brief paper, we shall focus on this second goal. Based on our studies of sensitization in *Aplysia*, we will examine first the interrelationships between two major types of memory — short-term, lasting minutes and hours, and long-term, lasting days and weeks. Then, we will explore the relationship between nonassociative and associative learning by comparing sensitization to classical conditioning.

To examine these questions, we have used the gill-withdrawal reflex, a simple defensive reflex in *Aplysia*. When the siphon or mantle shelf of an *Aplysia* is stimulated by light touch, the siphon, mantle shelf and the underlying gill contract vigorously and withdraw into the mantle cavity (Fig. 1). This reflex is analogous to a vertebrate

---

1 Howard Hughes Medical Institute and Center for Neurobiology and Behavior, Columbia University College of Physicians and Surgeons, 722 West 168th Street, New York, NY 10032, USA

Molecular Aspects of Neurobiology
(ed. by R. Levi Montalcini et al.)
© Springer-Verlag Berlin Heidelberg 1986

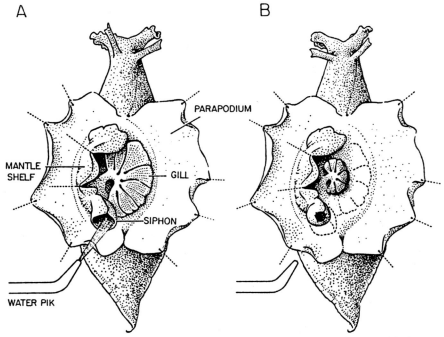

Fig. 1 A,B. Gill- and siphon-withdrawal reflex in *Aplysia: Top view* of *Aplysia* with the parapodia retracted to expose the gill and the mantle shelf. **A** Before the tactile stimulation (brief jet of water) to the siphon skin, the gill and the siphon are relayed. **B** After the stimulation, there is a brisk contraction of the gill and the siphon. The *dotted lines* indicate the relaxed position of the two organs

defensive escape or withdrawal response. This simple reflex can be modified by experience; it undergoes four types of learning: habituation, sensitization, classical conditioning, and operant conditioning (Pinsker et al. 1970–1973; Carew et al. 1983; Hawkins et al. 1985).

In this behavioral system, it is possible to examine learning at three levels: behavioral, cellular, and molecular. At the behavioral level we have attempted to characterize various forms of learning and obtain the time course for the short- and long-term memory of each form. At the cellular level, we are trying to specify, for each form, the locus of the physiological changes. Finally, we are using a variety of biochemical and cell biological approaches to specify, at the molecular level, the mechanisms of the plastic changes.

During the past ten years, we have applied behavioral, cellular, and molecular approaches to study the reflex system in vivo using semi-intact preparations or the isolated central nervous system. Recently, we have reduced and simplified the reflex further, using two in vitro systems. We have used a dissociated cell culture system developed in *Aplysia* by Schacher (Rayport and Schacher 1986) to reconstitute elementary components of the learning system. We have then used this reconstituted system to examine the relation of short-term to long-term sensitization. Finally, we

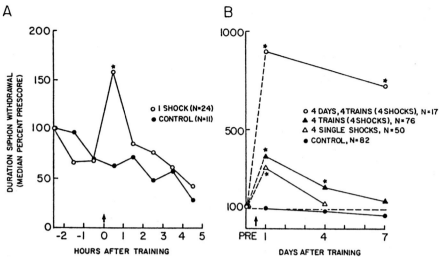

Fig. 2A,B. Short-term and long-term sensitization of the withdrawal reflex in *Aplysia*. A Time course of sensitization after a single strong electrical shock to the tail or the neck of the subject (*arrow*). The siphon withdrawal was tested once every 0.5 h and the mean of each two consecutive responses is shown. The experimental animals had significantly longer withdrawals than controls for more than 1 h. B Summary of different groups of animals receiving various amounts of stimulation. There is a gradual increase in the duration of long-term sensitization which is a function of the amount of training administered. Animals receiving four shocks (0.5 h intervals) showed a smaller effect than animals receiving four trains of four shocks. A much larger effect is observed if the four trains of four shocks is repeated for 4 consecutive days. *Asterisks* indicate points that are significantly different from control points. (From Frost et al. 1985)

have used a cell-free system to examine the molecular relationship of sensitization to classical conditioning.

2. On the Relation of Short-term to Long-term Sensitization

Sensitization is an elementary form of nonassociative learning in which an animal learns about the properties of a single, noxious (sensitizing) stimulus. The animal learns to strengthen its defensive reflexes and to respond vigorously to a variety of previously neutral or indifferent stimuli after it has been exposed to a potentially threatening or noxious stimulus. Sensitization training gives rise to both short- and long-term effects. A single training trial produces sensitization that lasts from minutes to hours. Repeated training trials prolong the enhancement of the reflex for days and even weeks (Pinsker et al. 1973; Frost et al. 1985; Fig. 2).

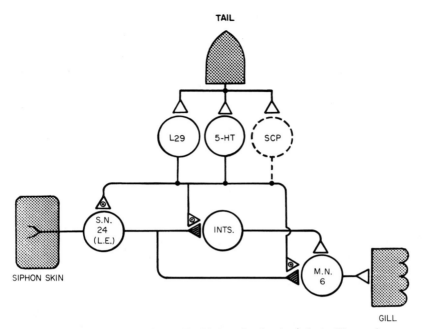

Fig. 3. Simplified diagram of the gill-withdrawal reflex in *Aplysia*. The mechanoreceptor neurons (*24*) carry the information from the siphon skin to interneurons and gill motor neurons (*6*). Stimulation of the tail (or the neck region) excites subsets of facilitator neurons which increase the synaptic transmission between the sensory neurons and their follower cells. Some facilitators may be serotonergic or peptidergic (*SCP*). The transmitter of the only identified facilitator group of interneurons (*L29* cluster) is not yet known

3. Short-term Sensitization Involves Covalent Modification of Pre-existing Proteins

The mantle shelf and the siphon are each innervated by a separate cluster of about 24 sensory cells, one located on the left side (the siphon or LE sensory neurons) and the other on the right side of the abdominal ganglion (the mantle or the RE sensory neurons). The sensory neurons from each cluster make excitatory monosynaptic connections with interneurons and motoneurons that produce the withdrawal reflex. We have primarily focused on the monosynaptic portion of the reflex circuit consisting of the sensory neurons, the motor neurons, and their connections. A sensitizing stimulus applied to the tail (or the neck region) activates facilitating neurons that act on the terminals of the sensory neurons to enhance transmitter release, by a process of presynaptic facilitation (Fig. 3).

We do not know yet many of the elements of the facilitatory system or the transmitters they utilize. But we have reason to believe that at least three sets of facilitator neurons are involved utilizing three transmitters: (1) serotonin, (2) two peptides SCP_A and SCP_B, and (3) the yet unidentified transmitter of the L29 facilitator neurons (Abrams et al. 1984b). All three simulate the effect of a sensitizing stimulus in the reflex. The L29 cells are identified but their transmitter is not. The L29 transmitter is thought to resemble serotonin because it is packaged in similar vesicles and because the L29 cells have a high affinity uptake system for serotonin (Bailey et al. 1983). In addition to the terminals from L29, immunocytochemical studies indicate that the sensory neurons are innervated by terminals containing serotonin and the SCPs. Mackey and Hawkins have recently begun to localize and identify the cell bodies of the serotonergic neurons that end on the sensory regions and to show that they can facilitate the sensory neurons. A similar search is still needed for the SCP containing nerve cells.

We will summarize here the work done with serotonin. But, as far as we can tell, all three transmitters have a common action — they trigger a cascade of events which are cAMP-mediated and lead to increased synaptic transmission.

Based upon electrophysiological, voltage-clamp, patch clamp, and biochemical experiments, we have suggested a molecular model for presynaptic facilitation (for review see Kandel and Schwartz 1982). According to this model, serotonin and other transmitters released by the facilitating neurons activate a transmitter-sensitive adenylate cyclase in the membrane of the presynaptic terminals of the sensory neurons that increases cyclic AMP content within these terminals (Fig. 4). Cyclic AMP then activates a protein kinase that phosphorylates a special K^+ channel protein or a protein that is associated with it (Shuster et al. 1985). This phosphorylation reduces the K^+ current that normally contributes significantly to the repolarization of the action potential. Reduction of this K^+ current prolongs the action potential and allows more Ca^{2+} to flow into the terminals and more transmitter is released. In addition, protein phosphorylation modulates the buffering of Ca^{2+} within the cell. Consequently more transmitter can be mobilized for release (Hochner et al. 1985). Both of these processes seem only to involve covalent modification (phosphorylation) of pre-existing proteins; short-term memory does not require the synthesis of new proteins (Schwartz et al. 1971; Montarolo et al. 1985).

4. A Beginning Analysis of Long-term Sensitization

How is this short-term form of memory related to the long-term form? Do they represent distinct processes with different loci and different mechanisms or different phases of a single process?

As early as 1890 William James first suggested that there may be different processes forming short- and long-term memories. Many subsequent studies in animals and humans confirmed James' observation and illustrated that newly formed memories are susceptible to disruption for a short period of time after formation, whereas later memories become more stable and less capable of being disrupted. Following this early work, there were repeated attempts to determine whether these two apparently different forms of memory represent separate processes or merely two different phases of a single process. The conflict between the one- and two-process models is central to the renewed interest that psychologists have shown in the neural analysis of learning, and poses a specific challenge to the cellular analysis of memory processes (Davis and Squire 1984).

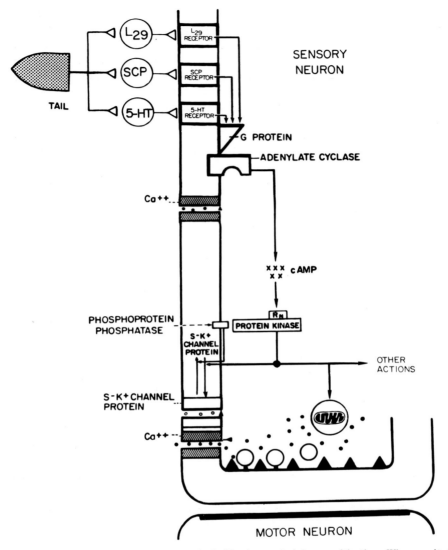

Fig. 4. Molecular model of presynaptic facilitation underlying sensitization. When excited, the various groups of facilitator neurons activate a sequence of events which led to a cAMP-dependent phosphorylation of substrate proteins which results in the closure of a special K channel and in a change in the Ca^{2+} buffering in the presynaptic terminals of the sensory neuron. The resulting increase in duration of the action potential leads to an increase of Ca^{2+} current. This effect together with the increase in the free Ca^{2+} in the terminals result in a greater synaptic transmission

A first step in the analysis of long-term memory in our system was recently achieved by Frost et al. (1985). They asked the following questions: Is the locus that is involved in the short-term sensitization also modulated in the long-term sensitization? They measured the amplitude of the monosynaptic EPSPs between sensory neurons and the gill motor neuron L7 in a group of sensitized animals and a control group of animals. They found that the monosynaptic connection between the sensory neurons and identified cell L7 that is facilitated during the short-term process is also facilitated during long-term sensitization.

Does this long-term change involve a morphological change? With this question in mind, Bailey and Chen (1983) have visualized the sensory neuron terminals directly using HRP, and analyzed the changes in the number and distribution of the synaptic vesicles and in the size and extent of the active zones. They compared the frequency of active zones in sensory neuron varicosities of control and sensitized animals. They found that in sensitized animals a larger percentage of varicosities had an active zone. The mean ratio of active zones to varicosities increased from 41% in control animals to 65% in long-term sensitized animals. Moreover, the total surface membrane area of sensory neuron active zones and the total number of vesicles associated with each release site were also increased.

The results of Bailey and Chen (1983) suggest that active zones are plastic structures and that learning may modulate these sites to alter synaptic effectiveness. These morphological changes could represent an anatomical substrate for the consolidation of long-term memory.

5. Reconstitution of Short- and Long-term Synaptic Plasticity in Dissociated Cell Culture

Recently Rayport and Schacher (1986) have succeeded in reconstituting part of the neuronal circuit mediating the gill-withdrawal reflex in dissociated cell cultures. They have cocultured dissociated sensory cells and a motor cell (L7). After 3 days in tissue culture, the chemical synaptic transmission is restored between the sensory neurons and the motor cell. As in vivo, the monosynaptic connection undergoes short-term facilitation when treated with 5-HT, SCP$_B$, or the L29 transmitter. Since long-term sensitization can be produced in the intact animal by presenting four or more facilitating stimuli at regular intervals, we have used an analogous protocol in the dissociated culture (five repeated brief exposure to 1 μM 5-HT, each separated by 15 min) to produce long-term facilitation. The amplitude of the EPSP's was measured before treatment with 5-HT and 24 h later. We found a significant change in EPSP amplitudes of the 5-HT treated cultures, whereas in control untreated cultures there was none (Montarolo et al. 1985).

To determine whether this long-lasting facilitation is dependent on synthesis of new proteins, we are currently using this culture system, as well as the isolated abdominal ganglion, to study the effect of inhibitors of protein and RNA synthesis. In preliminary experiments, we used anisomycin (10 μm) which blocks protein synthesis by more than 90%. Anisomycin is added to cultures 30 min before starting the training protocol with 5-HT and is then kept in the cultures until 1 h after the last 5-HT application. With this protocol, we have found that anisomycin blocks the 5-HT-induced long-term increase of EPSP amplitudes without interfering with short-term facilitation.

These results suggest that long- and short-term memory can be pharmacologically dissociated. Learning initiates two memory traces acting on a common locus (the monosynaptic connection between the sensory and motor neurons), but it appears to do so using different molecular mechanisms. Short-term memory results from a covalent, posttranslational modification (phosphorylation) of existing proteins; long-term memory may require the synthesis of new proteins.

6. On the Relationship of Sensitization to Classical Conditioning

Whereas sensitization involves an animal learning about the properties of a single stimulus, in classical conditioning, the animal learns about the relationship between two stimuli. Classical conditioning involves the selective enhancement of one reflex pathway when the stimulus for that pathway (the CS) is repeatedly paired with a reinforcing stimulus (the US) so that the CS comes to signal and predict the US. When an animal has been conditioned, it has learned that the conditioned stimulus (CS) predicts the unconditioned stimulus (US). Thus, in Pavlov's classical experiment, the dog salivates in response to the bell because it has learned that the bell predicts food. In contrast, nonassociative learning such as sensitization does not require temporal pairing of stimuli and does not teach the animal to associate a relationship between the two stimuli.

Often a reflex can be modified by sensitization as well as by classical conditioning. In those cases, the response enhancement produced by classical conditioning has three features that distinguish it from sensitization: (1) Classical conditioning produces greater and longer lasting enhancement than that produced by sensitization. (2) Whereas the consequences of sensitization are broad and affect a range of defensive responses, the effects of classical conditioning are exquisitely specific and enhance only those responses whose stimuli are paired with the US. Finally, (3) classical conditioning exhibits exquisite temporal specificity. Each of these three features occurs in the gill- and siphon-withdrawal reflex in *Aplysia* (Carew et al. 1983; Fig. 5).

7. Sensitization and Classical Conditioning Share Aspects of the Same Mechanisms

Hawkins et al. (1983) have found that classical conditioning of the withdrawal reflex involves a pairing-specific enhancement of presynaptic facilitation. They have called this type of enhancement *activity-dependent amplification of presynaptic facilitation*. Similar results have been obtained independently by Walters and Byrne (1983), who have found activity-dependent synaptic facilitation in identified sensory neurons that

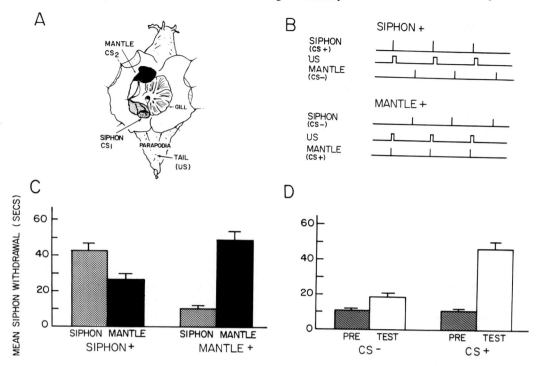

MEAN SIPHON WITHDRAWAL (SECS)

Fig. 5A–D. Differential conditioning of the defensive withdrawal reflex. **A** Dorsal view of *Aplysia* illustrating the two sites used to deliver conditioned stimuli: the siphon and the mantle shelf. The US was an electric shock delivered to the tail. For illustrative purposes, the parapodia are shown intact and retracted; however, the behavioral studies were all carried out in freely moving animals whose parapodia had been surgically removed. **B** Paradigm for differential conditioning: one group (*Siphon +*) received siphon CS (*CS+*) paired with US and the mantle CS (*CS-*) specifically unpaired with the US; the other group (*Mantle +*) received the mantle stimulus as CS+ and the siphon stimulus as CS-. The intertrial interval was 5 min. **C** Results of an experiment using the paradigm of (**B**). Testing was carried out 30 min after 15 training trials. The Siphon+ group (n = 12) showed significantly greater response (p < 0.05) to the siphon CS than to the mantle CS, whereas the Mantle+ group (n = 12) showed significantly greater response (p < 0.01) to the mantle CS than to the siphon CS. **D** Pooled data from (**C**). Test scores from the unpaired (*CS-*) and paired (*CS+*) pathways are compared to their respective pretest scores. The CS+ test scores are significantly greater than the CS- test scores (p < 0.005), demonstrating that differential conditioning has occurred. (From Carew et al. 1983)

innervate the tail of *Aplysia*. Because in classical conditioning the CS precedes the US, the sensory neurons of the CS pathway are set into activity and fire action potentials just before the facilitator neurons of the US pathway become active. When action potentials are generated in a sensory neuron just before the US is delivered, the US produces substantially more facilitation of the synaptic potential than if the US is not paired with activity in the sensory neuron. *Thus, at least aspects of the mechanism for the temporal specificity of classical conditioning occur within the sensory neuron itself.* The pairing specificity characteristic of classical conditioning results because the presynaptic facilitation is augmented or amplified by temporally paired spike activity in the sensory neurons.

What are the molecular mechanisms for presynaptic facilitation and its enhancement by activity? Both Abrams et al. (1984a) and Ocorr et al. (1985) have found that classical conditioning produces an amplification of the cAMP cascade which underlies the synaptic facilitation during sensitization. Cells that have just been active prior to the application of 5-HT show a greater increase of cAMP than those that are not active or that are active in an unpaired fashion.

Which aspect of activity in a sensory neuron interacts with the process of presynaptic facilitation to amplify the cAMP cascade? This question has two parts: (a) What signal from the action potential serves to amplify presynaptic facilitation and the cyclic AMP cascade? and (b) What component of the cascade recognizes the signal? We have obtained evidence that at least part of the signal for activity is given by the influx of Ca^{2+} with each action potential. In the absence of Ca^{2+}, pairing does not produce activity-dependent facilitation (Abrams et al. 1983). Similarly, the activity-dependent effect is blocked if a cell is injected with EGTA. Thus, our findings indicate that whereas 5-HT and the other facilitating transmitters act as the signal for the US, Ca^{2+} acts as the signal for the CS and accounts for the temporal specificity of classical conditioning.

Where do the two signals converge? Where does Ca^{2+} exert its action? To explore this question, Abrams and Kandel (1985) have recently developed a cellular homogenate preparation containing sensory neurons. They asked which component of the cascade accounts for the greater increase of cAMP observed during classical conditioning. Is the degradative enzyme (the phosphodiesterase) depressed, or is the synthetic enzyme (the cyclase) stimulated? Increasing Ca^{2+} did not depress the phosphodiesterase, but it did increase both the basal cyclase activity and the ability of 5-HT to stimulate the cyclase.

Adenylcyclase is a complex enzyme consisting of a receptor protein to which hormones bind, two (or more) regulatory subunits and a catalytic subunit. The catalytic subunits exist in two forms. Many cells have a catalytic unit that does not require Ca^{2+} for its activation. But nerve cells and certain others have a second form that is stimulated by Ca^{2+} via the calcium binding protein, calmodulin. *Aplysia's* nervous system contains the species of cyclase that is stimulated by Ca^{2+} calmodulin.

We think that Ca^{2+} influx interacts with the action of serotonin on the level of the Ca^{2+}/calmodulin-dependent adenylate cyclase, because in the presence of Ca^{2+}/comodulin, this cyclase responds more effectively to serotonin. Our data suggest that the Ca^{2+} calmodulin-dependent adenylate cyclase may be an important convergence point for classical conditioning. It is here that the influence of the CS (the Ca^{2+} influx) and the influence of the US (the serotonin-activation of the adenyl cyclase) interact (Fig. 6).

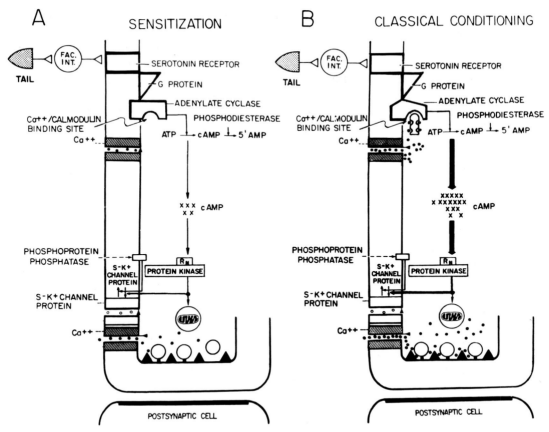

Fig. 6A,B. Hypothetical model suggesting how allosteric properties of the Ca^{2+}/calmodulin-dependent adenylate cyclase may account for the association mechanisms of classical conditioning in *Aplysia*. **A** Sensitization. In the absence of spike activity and Ca^{2+} influx in the sensory neuron, the facilitating transmitter released by the US is shown producing a modest activation of the cyclase, stimulating a small amount of cAMP synthesis. The Ca^{2+} channel is shown closed and calmodulin is shown without Ca^{2+} bound. **B** Classical conditioning. CS precedes US. The CS has caused spike activity in the sensory neuron, thereby transiently opening Ca^{2+} channels and allowing Ca^{2+} influx. Ca^{2+}/calmodulin is shown binding to adenylate cyclase. If the US occurs during this period of calmodulin activation, stimulation of the cyclase is shown to be potentiated, causing a greater synthesis of cAMP

8. An Overall View

In conclusion, we would make four additional points:

1. It may now be possible to explore in molecular detail the relationship between short- and long-term memory. Our preliminary data suggest that even though the two processes share a number of features, they differ from one another in terms of molecular mechanisms. Thus, short-term memory involves covalent modifications of pre-

existing proteins, whereas long-term memory seems to involve new protein synthesis and perhaps alterations in gene expression.

2. Our evidence shows that classical conditioning and sensitization are not distinctly different processes as earlier behavioral experiments had suggested. Rather, when analyzed on the cellular level, these two forms of learning are found to share components of a common molecular cascade. This conclusion has also now been supported by the independent work of William Quinn and his colleagues (Quinn and Greenspan 1984), using genetic approaches in *Drosophila*, as well as by Walters and Burne (1983) in *Aplysia*. Perhaps most dramatically, work on *Drosophila* has shown that a single common genetic defect in mutants disrupts both sensitization and classical conditioning.

3. A corollary to this finding is the interesting possibility that there may be a molecular alphabet for learning whereby more complex processes, such as the higher-order forms, would utilize components of the molecular machinery involved in simple forms of learning. If this building-block model proves true, we may expect our understanding of learning to progress somewhat more rapidly in the future than it has in the past.

4. Studies in both *Drosophila* and *Aplysia* illustrate a point which initially seemed worrisome. How can learning, a very special form of cellular regulation, use a universal regulatory system such as the cAMP cascade? The answer lies in several parts. First of all, even though most cells have the machinery of the cAMP cascade, learning clearly derives a major part of its complexity from the specificity of the connections made by the CS and US, so that the wiring interconnects certain cells and not others. Second, some cells and not others will have an adenylate cyclase coupled to a particular transmitter receptor in their plasma membrane. Third, as the data in *Aplysia* and *Drosophila* illustrate, the detailed expression of the cAMP cascade can vary dramatically from cell to cell. For example, there are many substrate proteins of the cAMP-dependent kinase, but only some will be present in a particular cell. Conversely, of the four K^+ channels present in the sensory neurons, only one is affected by a cAMP-dependent kinase. Finally, the four major enzymes in the cAMP cascade (cyclase, kinase, phosphodiesterase and phosphatase) exist in multiple (isozymic) forms. Different cells may utilize different combinations of these enzymatic forms.

These considerations also explain why *Drosophila* mutants such as *dunce* and *rutabaga* − which all have gross biochemical defects in cyclic AMP metabolism, are nonetheless behaviorally normal except in tests that look at behavioral plasticity. One might have expected that the flies with the major defect in an important enzyme, such as phosphodiesterase or adenylcyclase, would be dead; instead they are practically normal. In both *dunce* and *rutabaga*, however, even though one enzyme seems to be completely missing, it is one of at least two forms of the same enzyme. Perhaps the two mutants are missing the most dispensible form of the enzyme − perhaps one particularly concerned with behavioral plasticity. Thus, there may be isoenzymes within the cyclic AMP cascade which represents subpopulations of enzymes which are specifically relevant to the machinery for memory. The work of Schwartz and his colleagues (1983) on regulatory subunits of kinase also supports this idea. Put another way, the capability of learning seems to be grafted upon a common regulatory cascade. A few additional isozymes and substrate proteins may allow the cAMP cascade to be modified by experience in an activity-dependent way.

Acknowledgment. The authors are grateful for the support of the European Molecular Biology Organisation (P.M.) and the McKnight Foundation.

References

Abrams TW, Kandel ER (1985) Roles of calcium and adenylate cyclase in activity-dependent facilitation, a cellular mechanism for classical conditioning in *Aplysia*. J Neurochem 44:512

Abrams TW, Carew TJ, Hawkins RD, Kandel ER (1983) Aspects of the cellular mechanisms of temporal specificity in conditioning in *Aplysia:* Preliminary evidence for Ca^{++} influx as a signal of activity. Soc Neurosci Abstr 9:168

Abrams TW, Bernier L, Hawkins RD, Kandel ER (1984a) Possible roles of Ca^{2+} and cAMP in activity-dependent facilitation, a mechanism for associative learning in *Aplysia*. Soc Neurosci Abstr 10:269

Abrams TW, Castellucci VF, Camardo JS, Kandel ER, Lloyd PE (1984b) Two endogenous neuropeptides modulate the gill- and siphon-withdrawal reflex in *Aplysia* by presynaptic facilitation involving cAMP-dependent closure of a serotonin-sensitive potassium channel. Proc Natl Acad Sci USA 81:7956–7960

Bailey CH, Chen M (1983) Morphological basis of long-term habituation and sensitization in *Aplysia*. Science 220:91–93

Bailey CH, Hawkins RD, Chen M (1983) Uptake of (^{3}H) serotonin in the abdominal ganglion of *Aplysia californica:* Further studies on the morphological and biochemical basis of presynaptic facilitation. Brain Res 272:71–81

Carew TJ, Hawkins RD, Kandel ER (1983) Differential classical conditioning of a defensive withdrawal reflex in *Aplysia californica*. Science 219:397–400

Davis HP, Squire LR (1984) Protein synthesis and memory: A review. Psychol Bull 96:518–559

Frost WN, Castellucci VF, Hawkins RD, Kandel ER (1985) The direct-synaptic connections from the sensory neurons participate in the storage of long-term memory for sensitization of the gill- and siphon-withdrawal reflex in *Aplysia*. (In press)

Hawkins RD, Abrams TW, Carew TJ, Kandel ER (1983) A cellular mechanism of classical conditioning in *Aplysia:* Activity-dependent amplification of presynaptic facilitation. Science 219:400–415

Hawkins RD, Clark GA, Kandel ER (1985) Operant conditioning and differential classical conditioning of gill withdrawal in *Aplysia*. Soc Neurosci Abstr 11 (in press)

Hochner B, Schacher S, Klein M, Kandel ER (1985) Presynaptic facilitation in *Aplysia* sensory neurons: A process independent of K^+ current modulation becomes important when transmitter release is depressed. Soc Neurosci Abstr 11 (in press)

Kandel ER, Schwartz JH (1982) Molecular biology of an elementary form of learning: Modulation of transmitter release by cyclic AMP. Science 218:433–443

Kandel ER, Abrams TW, Bernier L, Carew TJ, Hawkins RD, Schwartz JH (1983) Classical conditioning and sensitization share aspects of the same molecular cascade in *Aplysia*. Cold Spring Harbor Symp Quant Biol 48:821–830

Montarolo PG, Castellucci VF, Goelet P, Kandel ER, Schacher S (1985) Long-term facilitation of the monosynaptic connection between sensory neurons and motor neurons of the gill-withdrawal reflex in *Aplysia* in dissociated cell culture. Soc Neurosci Abstr 11:795

Ocorr KA, Walters ET, Byrne JH (1985) Associative conditioning analog selectively increases cAMP levels of tail sensory neurons in *Aplysia*. Proc Natl Acad Sci USA 82:2548–2552

Pinsker H, Kupfermann I, Castellucci VF, Kandel ER (1970) Habituation and dishabituation of the gill-withdrawal reflex in *Aplysia*. Science 167:1740–1742

Pinsker HM, Hening WA, Carew TJ, Kandel ER (1973) Long-term sensitization of a defensive withdrawal reflex in *Aplysia*. Science 182:1039–1042

Quinn WG, Greenspan RJ (1984) Learning and courtship in *Drosophila:* Two stories with mutants. Annu Rev Neurosci 7:67–93

Rayport SG, Schacher S (1986) Synaptic plasticity *in vitro:* Cell culture of identified *Aplysia* neurons mediating short-term habituation and sensitization. J Neurosci (in press)

Schwartz JH, Castellucci VF, Kandel ER (1971) Functions of identified neurones and synapses in abdominal ganglion of *Aplysia* in absence of protein synthesis. J Neurophysiol 34:939–953

Schwartz JH, Bernier L, Castellucci VF, Palazzolo M, Saitoh T, Stapleton A, Kandel ER (1983) What molecular steps determine the time course of the memory for short-term sensitization in *Aplysia?* Cold Spring Harbor Symp Quant Biol 48:811–819

Shuster MJ, Camardo JS, Siegelbaum SA, Kandel ER (1985) Cyclic AMP-dependent protein kinase closes the serotonin-sensitive K^+ channels of *Aplysia* sensory neurons in cell-free membrane patches. Nature 313:392–395

Walters ET, Byrne JH (1983) Associative conditioning of single sensory neurons suggests a cellular mechanism for learning. Science 219:405–408

Serotonin Modulates the Action Potential in Growth Cone Precursors of Sensory Neuron Terminals in *Aplysia*

F. BELARDETTI, S. SCHACHER, E.R. KANDEL, and S.A. SIEGELBAUM[1]

1. Introduction

Serotonin (5-HT) closes a specific class of K^+ channels in the sensory neurons of *Aplysia,* resulting in a slow EPSP, an increase in action potential duration (APD), and presynaptic facilitation of transmitter release (Klein and Kandel 1978, 1980; Kandel and Schwartz 1982; Siegelbaum et al. 1982). Because of the small size and inaccessibility of the sensory neuron terminals, previous studies have been limited to readings from the cell body of the sensory neurons. To explore whether K^+ channel closure also occurs in presynaptic terminals, we have used the patch clamp technique and studied the action of 5-HT on both intact and isolated growth cones (g.c.), the precursors to the mature synaptic terminal of *Aplysia* sensory neurons in culture.

2. Methods and Procedures

Pleural sensory cell bodies with their initial axon were plated in polylisine-coated dishes containing hemolymph, L15, salts, glutamine and antibiotics (Schacher and Proshansky 1983; Rayport and Schacher 1985). The cut end of the axon attached to the dish within 12–14 h, giving rise to a large, flat g.c. suitable for electrophysiological recordings.

3. Results

Patch pipettes filled with an "intracellular" solution (containing KCl, EGTA, MgATP, GTP and HEPES at pH 7.3) were sealed either against the soma or the growth cone. After breaking the patch of membrane underlying the pipette by applying suction, resting potentials of −50 mV to −60 mV could be recorded under current-clamp

---

1 College of Physicians & Surgeons of Columbia University, 722 West 168th Street, New York, NY 10032, USA

Molecular Aspects of Neurobiology
(ed. by Rita Levi Montalcini et al.)
© Springer-Verlag Berlin Heidelberg 1986

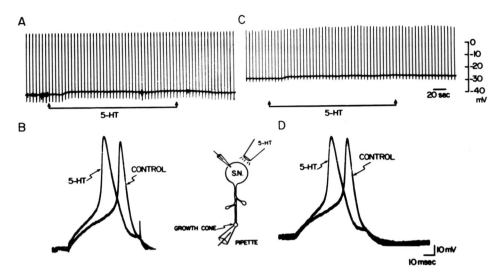

Fig. 1A—D. Effect of serotonin application on the resting potential and action potentials recorded from the cell bodies and growth cones of *Aplysia* sensory neurons in culture. **A, B** Recordings from cell body. **C, D** Show recordings from the growth cone. **A, C** Simultaneous records of membrane potential from chart recorder showing a small slow depolarization in response to 5-HT application to cell body (duration indicated by *bar*). Brief spikes are action potentials elicited by constant current pulses. **B, D** Superimposed action potentials at a faster sweep photographed from oscilloscope. 5-HT causes a 31% increase in AP duration in the cell body (**B**) and a 29% increase in the growth cone (**D**). The drawing (*inset*) depicts the experimental protocol

mode. Recordings from cell bodies show that a brief puff of 5-HT (1—100 μM serotonin creatine sulfate) to the cell body produces a slow depolarization of 4—10 mV, a 15—20% increase in the input resistance, and a 14—30% increase in APD duration (Fig. 1A,B).

Next we recorded from the intact g.c. (n = 4). A second electrode was inserted in the cell body, and used to monitor the soma potential and to inject current (Fig. 1). Action potentials fired in the cell body were conducted to the g.c. with a variable degree of attenuation. After application of 5-HT either on the g.c. or on the cell body, the g.c. membrane shows a slow depolarization of 2—7 mV (Fig. 1C), a 3—14% increase in input resistance, and a 25% increase in AP duration (Fig. 1D).

To determine whether these effects of 5-HT resulted from a modulation of ionic conductances within the growth cone itself, we have recorded from g.c.s that have been mechanically isolated from their axons with a glass needle. Most of the growth cones survived this procedure and depolarizing current pulses elicited action potentials. Direct application of 5-HT (n = 6) induced a slow 2—5 mV depolarization of the resting potential (Fig. 2B), and 11—22% broadening of the APD (Fig. 2C), and a 12—50% increase in input resistance. Application of a control solution (n = 2, creatinine sulfate in sea water) had no effect.

To understand the ionic mechanism underlying these changes in the g.c. membrane, we have begun to voltage-clamp the isolated growth cone. Holding the membrane

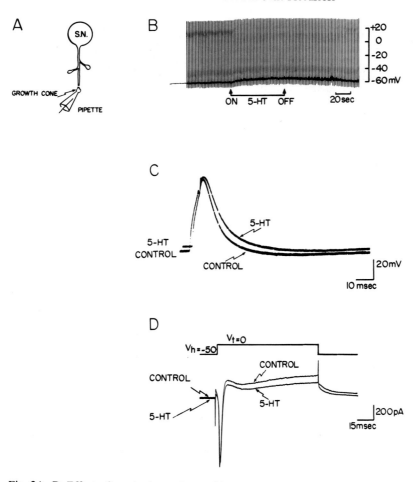

Fig. 2A–D. Effect of serotonin on the resting potential, action potential and ionic currents from an isolated growth cone. **A** Experimental protocol. **B** Slow chart recording of membrane potential showing slow depolarization with 5-HT. The *bar* marks the duration of serotonin application. **C** Two superimposed action potentials from oscilloscope at faster sweep before and after serotonin application. Action potential duration increased by 21% in response to 5-HT. **D** Superimposed voltage clamp current records in response to a depolarization from −50 mV to 0 mV. Pulse elicits a brief inward current followed by delayed outward current. 5-HT decreases net inward current at both holding potential and during depolarization

potential at −50 mV and applying 100 ms depolarizing test pulses above −20 mV elicited a fast activating and inactivating inward current that was followed by a more slowly activating outward current. Direct application of 5-HT (n = 2) induced an inward shift of the holding current and a more prominent reduction of the delayed outward current and of the outward tail currents (Fig. 2D).

4. Discussion

These findings show that the electrophysiological effects of 5-HT in the sensory neuron g.c. are similar to the effects produced in the cell body and suggest that the mechanism of AP broadening is not localized only to the cell body but occurs in nerve processes as well. This then strengthens the view that action potential broadening may contribute to presynaptic facilitation at the sensory neuron terminals.

References

Klein M, Kandel ER (1978) Presynaptic modulation of voltage-dependent Ca^{2+} current: Mechanism for behavioral sensitization in *Aplysia californica*. Proc Natl Acad Sci USA 75:3512–3516

Klein M, Kandel ER (1980) Mechanism of calcium current modulation underlying presynaptic facilitation and behavioral sensitization in *Aplysia*. Proc Natl Acad Sci USA 77:6912–6916

Kandel ER, Schwartz JH (1982) Molecular biology of an elementary form of learning: Modulation of transmitter release by cyclic AMP. Science 218:433–443

Rayport S, Schacher S (1986) Synaptic plasticity *in vitro:* Cell culture of identified *Aplysia* neurons mediating short-term habituation and sensitization. J Neurosci (in press)

Schacher S, Proshansky E (1983) Neutrite regeneration by *Aplysia* neurons in dissociated cell culture: Modulation by *Aplysia* hemolymph and the presence of the initial axonal segment. J Neurosci 3:2403–2413

Siegelbaum S, Camardo JS, Kandel Er (1982) Serotonin and cAMP close single K^+ channels in *Aplysia* sensory neurones. Nature 299:413–417

Serotonin and cAMP Mediate Plastic Changes in Swimming Activity of *Hirudo m*

M. BRUNELLI, G. DEMONTIS, and G. TRAINA[1]

The mechanisms of some short-term non-associative learning processes, such as habituation and sensitization (or dishabituation) have been analyzed in detail in the defensive withdrawal reflex of the gill and the siphon of *Aplysia*. It has been shown that behavioral sensitization results from heterosynaptic facilitation of transmitter output on the mechanosensory neurons of the abdominal ganglion that innervate the gill and the siphon. The facilitation of synaptic output between sensory and motor neuron is mediated by two sets of neurons so far identified as the L28 and L29 cells which take contacts with terminal branches of sensory neurons. Serotonin as well as peptide transmitters (small cardioactive peptides SCPa and SCPb) or other unknown transmitters converge to produce synaptic facilitation in the sensory neurons via different receptors triggering a common molecular chain of events to produce the same modulatory effect. The transmitter released activates an adenylate cyclase which increases the intracellular level of cAMP (Brunelli et al. 1976). This enhancement leads to a cAMP-dependent protein phosphorilation through a protein kinase activation which induces a suppression of a specific K^+ current. The block of K^+ current is thought to cause broadening of the presynaptic action potential and therefore a prolonged influx of Ca^{++} in the presynaptic terminal which potentiates the transmitter release (Kandel and Schwartz 1982).

Is this model of molecular cascade observed in *Aplysia* widespread along the phylogenetic scale? Do other alternative mechanisms exist? To address this question we have studied the mechanisms of short-term plastic changes in *Hirudo m*. Since many cellular networks of the leech segmental ganglia have been extensively investigated it appeared an advantageous model for a parallel study of short-term plasticity of the nervous system and changes in behavior. In each segmental ganglion it is possible to identify a fixed number of neurons. The most commonly studied cells are the mechanosensory neurons: T, P, N, which respond to light touch, pressure and nociceptive stimuli; two giant cells, or Retzius cells, and various motor neurons. We studied non-associative learning in two different behavioral activities: (1) the shortening reflex; (2) swimming. In previous experiments we have seen that short-term changes underlying sensitization of the shortening reflex are mediated by serotonergic neurons via the intracellular increase of a second messenger of the nucleotide type (Belardetti et al. 1982). More recently a useful behavioral model has been identified in swimming activity. The

---

1 Istituto di Fisiologia, Università di Pisa and Istituto di Neurofisiologia, CNR, Pisa, Italy

Molecular Aspects of Neurobiology
(ed. by Rita Levi Montalcini et al.)
© Springer-Verlag Berlin Heidelberg 1986

circuitry underlying the swimming activity of the leech is made up of a chain of swim-related neurons. Mechanosensory stimulation activates in each segmental ganglion swim-initiating cells, which in turn excite the pattern generating interneurons that impinge upon all the longitudinal and flattened muscles. The rhythm is sustained by positive reciprocal feedback between the swim-initiating and pattern-generating interneurons. Although it is not possible to draw an outline of the network, many details regarding the initiation and modulation of the basic swim pattern need to be determined. The ablation of cephalic ganglion relieves an inhibition upon the swimming activity; therefore, light tactile or electrical stimuli onto skin patches of the tail produce the swimming activity. Electrical stimuli repetitively applied 1/min produce a gradual increase in latency between the onset of the stimulus and the start of the swimming response (habituation). When a strong noxious stimulus is applied the delayed latency suddenly shortens. The effect lasts for 30–60 min. Since it has been demonstrated that 5HT raises the probability that an animal will swim, we performed experiments to verify whether 5HT might mediate such a decrease in latency.

In a first series of experiments we demonstrated that 5HT injection into the whole animal induces a marked shortening of the latency. In addition, it has been shown that the injection of serotonin-blocking agent methysergide blocks the shortening of latency after nociceptive stimulation, preventing the behavioral dishabituation. In order to know whether cAMP might be involved in such an effect, we worked out experiments of pretreatment with an adenylate cyclase blocking agent RMI. We observed that this substance is capable of blocking the reduction of latency by nociceptive stimulation or by 5HT application. More recently, we have observed that injections into the animals of 5HT lead to a distruction of almost all the serotonergic neurons. In this case nociceptive stimulation is ineffective in inducing behavioral sensitization. To investigate the molecular mechanisms of these behavioral changes in swim-triggering, we performed experiments at the cellular level focusing on the effect of 5HT on sensory neurons activity and on serotonergic giant cells.

In T sensory neuron, 5HT application produces a marked dose-dependent depression of the afterhyperpolarization (AH) which follows the firing discharge. This AH seems due to the activation of both a K conductance and an electrogenic pump.

The reduction of AH amplitude is also obtained from direct intracellular stimulation of serotonergic neurons Rz. Both intracellular injection of cAMP and application of forskolin (an adenylate cyclase activator) induce a clearcut depression of AH (Biondi et al. 1982).

Dopamine also produces reduction of AH, but the effect is abolished with high Ca and high Mg^{++} solutions. The effect seems to be specific since no changes in AH amplitude has been observed in the P and N neurons.

In conclusion, the plastic changes observed in the swimming activity of the leech show similar mechanisms to the *Aplysia* withdrawal reflex, a chain of events starting from neurotransmitters (5HT) to cAMP elevation, protein phosphorilation and gating of ionic channels, but differing in the site of action and in specific molecular steps.

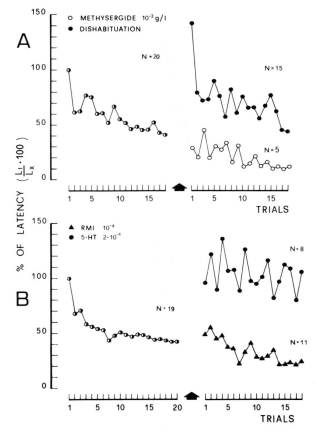

Fig. 1A,B. The graphs summarize the data on plastic changes in swim triggering activity. **A** In ordinate the percent of the reversal of the latency is depicted. 100% is the latency of the first trial. After repeated stimulation the latency increases (habituation). At the *arrow* a strong noxious stimulus is applied. A clearcut shortening of the latency occurs (*black dots*) (dishabituation). The *lower curve* (*white dots*) shows the block of the dishabituation after methysergide treatment. **B** After the habituation, application of 5HT induces a shortening of the latency (*black dots*) when the cyclase blocking agent RMI is applied the dishabituation is prevented (*black triangles*)

References

Belardetti F, Biondi C, Colombaioni L, Brunelli M, Trevisani A (1982) Role of serotonin and cyclic AMP on facilitation of the fast conducting system activity in the Hirudo medicinalis. Brain Res 246:89–103

Biondi C, Belardetti F, Brunelli M, Portolan A, Trevisani A (1982) Increased synthesis of cyclic AMP and short-term plastic changes in the segmental ganglia of the leech, Hirudo m. Cell Mol Neurobiol 2:81–91

Brunelli M, Castellucci V, Kandel ER (1976) Synaptic facilitation and behavioral sensitization in *Aplysia:* possible role of serotonin and cAMP. Science 194:1178–1181

Kandel ER, Schwartz JH (1982) Molecular biology of learning: modulation of transmitter release. Science 218:433–443

NGF Modulates the Synthesis of a Nuclear Lactic Dehydrogenase with Single-stranded DNA-Binding Properties

S. BIOCCA, A. CATTANEO, C. VOLONTÈ, and P. CALISSANO[1]

1. Introduction

It is a well-established and widely recognized notion that tumor cells have a particularly active glycolysis (Warburg 1967). This phenomenon is generally known as Warburg effect, in recognition of the scientist who first identified this process and described it in many papers: "Oxygen gas, the donor of energy in plants and animals, is dethroned in cancer cells and replaced by an energy-yielding reaction of the lowest living forms, namely a fermentation of glucose".

Although more than 50 years of biochemical work has established a relationship between energy metabolism and neoplastic cells, whether they are causally related has not yet been fully clarified.

Recent work performed by our group on the clonal cell line PC12 provided further evidence for this relationship and, at the same time, prospected the possible involvement of one of the enzymes of anaerobic glycolysis, namely lactic-dehydrogenase (LDM), in nuclear functions involving DNA in its unfolded state (Biocca et al. 1984; Calissano et al. 1985; Cattaneo et al. 1985). Thus, PC12 cells, in the presence of the protein nerve growth factor (Levi Montalcini 1965; Levi Montalcini and Angeletti 1968; Calisssano et al. 1984) undergo mitotic arrest and differentiate into sympathetic-like cells (Greene and Tischler 1976). During onset of this impressive phenotypic change, these cells exhibit a progressive metabolic shift from a typical, highly glycolizing tumor population, to normal cells oxidizing glucose in the Krebs cycle (Morelli et al. 1985). At the same time, probably via an action at the level of transcription, they progressively reduce the synthesis and total content of LDH (Biocca et al. 1984; Calissano et al. 1985). While these events are in keeping with the above-mentioned notion on energy metabolism in normal versus neoplastic cells, our previous demonstration (Calissano et al. 1985; Biocca et al. 1984) that LDH binds selectively to single-stranded DNA, together with the finding that a large portion of LDH is found in the nuclear compartment associated to DNAse-sensitive structure (Cattaneo et al. 1985) points to a possible link between nuclear function of the cell and enzymes involved in glycolysis.

1 Istituto di Biologia Cellulare, CNR, Via Romagnosi 18/A, 00196 Rome, Italy

Molecular Aspects of Neurobiology
(ed. by Rita Levi Montalcini et al.)
© Springer-Verlag Berlin Heidelberg 1986

Table 1. Properties of lactic dehydrogenase, single-stranded DNA-binding protein (LDH-ssb)

Molecular weight in SDS electrophoresis	34.000
Isoelectric point	8.1 ± 0.2
Enzymatic activity	470 u/mg protein
In vitro binding to double-stranded DNA	no
Binding to single-stranded DNA	yes

2. Results

Analysis of the polypeptides synthesized in PC12 cells before (PC12−) and after (PC12+) incubation with NGF, revealed that synthesis of a 34K dalton protein representing 0.5−1.0% of total soluble proteins was virtually suppressed in PC12+ (Biocca et al. 1984). It was also found that this 34K dalton protein could be isolated in an almost pure form by affinity chromatography on single-stranded DNA (ss-DNA). On the basis of its high affinity for ssDNA, a simpler procedure was subsequently devised for the isolation of this polypeptide from different samples at a time. With this method, it was found that onset of mitotic arrest of PC12 cells induced by NGF paralleled inhibition of the synthesis of the 34K protein, while its breakdown was unaffected (Calissano et al. 1985). We also demonstrated that NGF-induced inhibition of the synthesis is probably achieved at the transcriptional level since mRNA for 34K protein is lowered in concomitance with reduction of the total content of the protein.

Analysis of the possible function of the 34K protein led to the surprising discovery that this polypeptide has lactic dehydrogenase (LDH) activity comparable to that of the enzyme purified from rabbit skeletal muscle, hence the definition of LDH-ssb for this protein (Calissano et al. 1985). Further studies along this line of investigation, based on peptide-mapping analysis and immunological studies with antibodies against LDH-ssb and rabbit muscle LDH, unequivocally confirmed that the two proteins have marked structural and functional homologies. The major physico-chemical properties of LDH-ssb are summarized in Table 1. Figure 1 demonstrates that the synthesis of LDH-ssb is 30-fold stimulated in lymphocytes undergoing lectin-induced blast transformation. This finding, together with our previous demonstration that synthesis of LDH-ssb protein is reduced in PC12+ cells, further stresses the close relationship between content and/or activity of this enzyme and the proliferative state of either normal or neoplastic cells. As mentioned in the introduction, however, a close correlation between glycolysis and proliferative state has been known for a long time. The finding that one of the enzymes of this pathway, i.e. LDH, specifically binds to ssDNA, as well as subsequent experiments to be reported below, added a new perspective to the possible function of LDH, especially in relationship to nuclear functions and proliferative activity of the cell.

As seen in Fig. 2, when antibodies against the LDH-ssb purified from PC12 cells are employed in indirect immunofluorescence studies, they reveal a strong staining which is confined to the nuclear compartment with the exception of nucleoli. We found that such staining is progressively, although not completely, abolished when

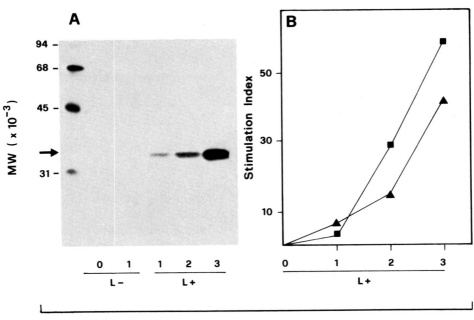

Fig. 1. Synthesis of LDH-ssb in lectin-stimulated spleen lymphocytes. LDH-ssb protein was isolated with the procedure described, from spleen lymphocytes incubated for different times in the absence ($L-$) or in the presence ($L+$) of Concanavalin A and Phythohaemoagglutinin and pulse-labeled for 2 h with ^{35}S-methionine. Sister cultures were labeled for 1 h with ^{3}H-thymidine. A-Electrophoretic pattern of the purified LDH-ssb. The radioactivity in the band was measured and is reported in B (▲—▲) which also shows the thymidine incorporation (■—■). Stimulation index refers to the fold increase of radioactive incorporation of the corresponding value obtained in the absence of lectins

cells, before fixation, are digested with DNAse indicating that a large portion of anti-LDH-ssb cross-reacting material is probably associated to chromatin structures (Cattaneo et al. 1985).

Experiments conducted at the E.M. with IgG-associated colloidal gold particles, confirmed the nuclear localization of LDH-ssb and demonstrated, as expected for a glycolytic enzyme, that LDH is also present in the cytoplasm. The reason for the exclusive nuclear localization, revealed through indirect immunofluorescence studies, is probably to be found in the existence of two different LDH-ssb pools: one is tightly associated (nuclear pool) and does not leak out during paraformaldehyde fixation before indirect staining, while the cytoplasmic pool is lost during this procedure due to its soluble, loosely bound distribution in the cytosol. On the contrary, glutar-aldehyde fixation for E.M. studies also cross-links the cytoplasmic pool and allows its detection (for a discussion of these findings see Cattaneo et al. 1985).

We have developed several monoclonal antibodies (m-ab) directed against different epitopes of LDH-ssb and employed them to probe its distribution within the nuclear

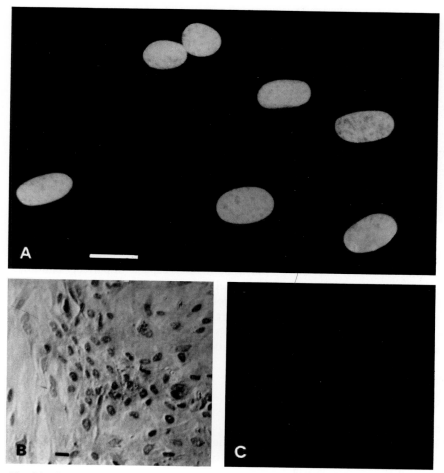

Fig. 2A−C. Indirect immunofluorescence staining with anti-LDH-ssb protein antibodies. Primary cultures of rat glial cells were fixed with 3.5% paraformaldehyde in PBS and permeabilized with Triton X-100 and incubated with immune (**A**) and preimmune (**C**) mouse serum. **B** Shows a representative field of the same type of cells stained with Coomassie blue. Scale bars represent 10 μm

compartment. These m-abs were specifically selected in order to identify LDH in different cytoplasmic or nuclear structures. As can be seen in Fig. 3 one of these, named S1D7, reveals a speckled distribution of LDH-ssb. This latter is somewhat similar to that revealed with antibodies directed against ribo nucleo protein particles.

If, then, a portion of LDH or a cross-reacting material is present within the nuclear compartment, one may wonder what is its function and if there are metabolic conditions, possibly connected with energy metabolism, that may modulate its nuclear presence in association to chromatin structures. While we have currently no answer to the first question, we have obtained some findings that may give a clue to the

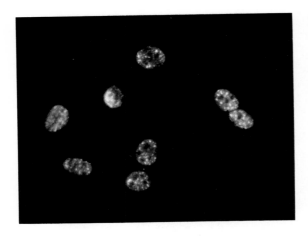

Fig. 3. Indirect immunofluorescence staining with m-ab S1D7. Primary cultures of rat glial cells were fixed as described in Fig. 2 and stained with monoclonal antibody S1D7 directed against LDH-ssb protein

second. As shown in Fig. 4, binding of LDH-ssb to ssDNA is fully inhibited by NADH at concentrations higher than 20–50 μM while NAD^+ is capable of partially inhibiting binding only at two orders of magnitude higher concentrations. We found that among many other nucleotides tested at 1.0 mM concentrations (AMP, ADP, ATP, GTP, CTP) only NADH inhibits binding demonstrating the specificity of interaction of LDH-ssb for ssDNA. These studies point to this essential component of energy metabolism as the possible modulator of such interaction.

3. Discussion

As mentioned in the introduction, while the correlation between high anaerobic glycolysis and active proliferation, especially of neoplastic cells, is well established, its functional significance is still matter of speculation. The finding reported in this article add some new facets to this controversial problem. Thus, an enzyme of anaerobic glycolysis largely represented in all tumors and rapidly growing cells, whereby it may constitute up to 1–2% of total soluble proteins, is found in the nuclear compartment, associated to chromatin and probably to other nuclear structures. Furthermore, synthesis of this enzyme and total content markedly decrease in the neoplastic PC12 cells in coincidence with mitotic arrest while strongly increasing in lectin-stimulated spleen lymphocytes. It is tempting to speculate that these findings are related and that LDH plays some important, as yet unidentified, role(s) in nuclear functions of neoplastic or normal cells. This role must be strictly connected with the specific tendency of LDH to interact with DNA in its unfolded state. Since, however, several crucial properties and functions (replication, transcription, recombination) are connected with the open structure of DNA, it is not possible, at present, even to postulate a precise role of LDH within this context. We may anticipate, on the basis of in vitro studies, that interaction of this enzyme with ssDNA regions can be modulated by the cellular content of NADH. It is worth considering, in this connection, that this nucleo-

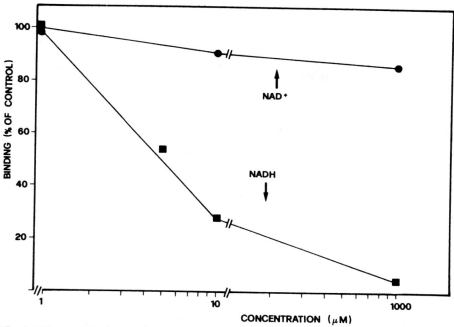

Fig. 4. Effect of *NAD*⁺ and *NADH* on the binding of LDH-ssb protein to ssDNA cellulose. Binding of LDH-ssb protein was performed as described (Calissano et al. 1985) in the presence of the indicated concentration of the nucleotides. After incubation of the PC12 extracts with dsDNA and ssDNA and elution with 2M NaCl from ssDNA the labeled proteins were electrophoresed and autoradiographed. The band corresponding to the LDH-ssb protein was cut and the radioactivity measured

tide, as well as some other coenzymes and high energy compounds such as ATP or GTP, undergo marked cellular fluctuations in their content in relationship with the functional state of normal or neoplastic cells (Hess et al. 1971).

Such oscillations are of large amplitude, up to two orders of magnitude above or below the average concentration, and can be induced by a rapid rise in the concentration of a substance like glucose or other compounds linked to energy metabolism. A protein like LDH may subserve the double, interrelated function of participating in glycolysis with its cytoplasmic pool and, at the same time, of transferring the information on the cellular ratio of NAD⁺/NADH, which in turn is directly coupled to energy metabolism, to portions of DNA in its unfolded state. According to this hypothesis, LDH would be bound to DNA when this ratio is high while it is free in the nuclear compartment when the ratio is low, i.e., when NADH is capable of competing with ssDNA for LDH. The precise nuclear function(s) modulated by this interplay remains to be established.

Acknowledgments. This work has been supported with grant n° 1-848 from March of Dimes and with grant Progetto Finalizzato Oncologia to P.C.

References

Biocca S, Cattaneo A, Calissano P (1984) Nerve growth factor inhibits the synthesis of a single-stranded DNA binding protein in pheochromocytoma cells (clone PC12). Proc Natl Acad Sci USA 81:2080–2084

Calissano P, Cattaneo A, Aloe L, Levi-Montalcini R (1984) The nerve growth factor (NGF). In: Li CH (ed) Hormonal proteins and peptides, vol 12. Academic, New York, pp 1–47

Calissano P, Volontè C, Biocca S, Cattaneo A (1985) Synthesis and content of a DNA binding protein with LDH activity are reduced by NGF in the neoplastic cell line PC12. Exp Cell Res 161: 117–128

Cattaneo A, Biocca S, Corvaja N, Calissano P (1985) Nuclear localization of a lactic dehydrogenase with single-stranded DNA binding properties. Exp Cell Res 161:130–140

Greene LA, Tischler A (1976) Establishment of a noradrenergic clonal line of rat adrenal pheochromocytoma cells which respond to nerve growth factor. Proc Natl Acad Sci USA 73:2424–2428

Hess B, Boiteux A (1971) Oscillatory phenomena in biochemistry. Annu Rev Biochem 40:237–258

Levi Montalcini R (1965) The nerve growth factor: its mode of action on sensory and sympathetic ganglia. Harvey Lect 60:217–259

Levi Montalcini R, Angeletti RU (1968) Nerve growth factor. Physiol Rev 48:534–569

Morelli S, Grasso M, Calissano P (1986) Effect of NGF on glucose utilization and nucleotides content of PC12 cells. J Neuroch (in press)

Warburg O (1967) The prime cause and prevention of cancer. Triltsch, Würzburg, Germany, pp 6–16

Molecular Cloning of a Gene Sequence Induced by NGF in PC12 Cells

A. LEVI, J.D. ELDRIDGE, and B.M. PATERSON[1]

Using a differential hybridization technique to screen a cDNA library constructed with mRNA from PC12 (Green and Tischler 1976) cells treated with nerve growth factor (NGF) (Levi Montalcini 1966), we have characterized a cDNA clone, VGF8a, corresponding to a mRNA induced to high levels as an early response to NGF. Preliminary experiments suggest that the expression of such a mRNA is tissue specific and is restricted to nerve cells.

Dose response studies indicate that half a maximum stimulation of the VGF8a RNA is induced by approximately 50 ng/ml of NGF, in good agreement with the published value of the Km of the NGF receptor (Calissano and Shelansky 1980). Time course experiments indicate that the level of the VGF8a transcript in PC12 cells is increased about 50-fold after 3 h of treatment with NGF and reaches a maximum within 5 h. Expression of the VGF8a sequence continues at high levels even after the cells have terminally differentiated. The amount of the VGF8a RNA in induced cells is comparable to that of actin as judged by the intensity of the hybridization signal on Northern blots. This finding is in good agreement with the frequency of cDNA clones hybridizing with VGF8a in the cDNA library from the NGF-induced PC12 cells. Moreover, in vitro translation products of mRNA hybrid selected by the VGF8a clone and a rat actin clone give bands of comparable intensity. It is not clear to us why in vivo studies have been unable to detect the protein corresponding to VGF8a sequence in the class of the abundant proteins (Garrels and Schubert 1979; McGuire and Greene 1978). One possibility is that the primary translation product of VGF8a (a 90,000 dalton polypeptide) is modified, processed, secreted, or compartmentalized (Biocca et al. 1983) so as to escape analysis on a two dimensional gels of the total cell proteins. Alternately, a rapid turnover of the protein or an inefficient translation of the mRNA, may result in the underrepresentation of the VGF8a coded protein with respect to its RNA. We hope to be able to elucidate this point by subcloning the VGF8a cDNA into expression vectors to obtain antibodies against the protein. A preliminary survey of different rat tissues and cell lines by Northern analysis suggests the VGF8a is expressed only in a subpopulation of the brain cells. It would be of great interest if the VGF8a mRNA is developmentally regulated in the brain in response to NGF-like factors.

1 Laboratory of Biochemistry, National Cancer Institute, National Institutes of Health, Bethesda, MD 20205, USA

Molecular Aspects of Neurobiology
(ed. by Rita Levi Montalcini et al.)
© Springer-Verlag Berlin Heidelberg 1986

Using the VGF8a cDNA as a probe we have isolated three independent recombinant phages by screening about four genomic equivalents from a rat genomic library. We are now in the process of characterizing the gene corresponding to the VGF8a cDNA clone.

References

Biocca S, Cattaneo A, Calissano P (1983) EMBO J 2:643
Calissano P, Shelansky ML (1980) Neuroscience 5:1033
Garrels JI, Schubert D (1971) J Biol Chem 254:7978
Green LA, Tischler AS (1976) Natl Acad Sci USA 73:2424
Levi Montalcini R (1966) Harvey Lect 60:217
McGuire JC, Greene LA (1978) Cell 15:357

Thymocytes as Potential Target Cells for Nerve Growth Factor

A. CATTANEO[1]

Nerve Growth Factor (NGF) is the best characterized protein regulating development in the nervous system (Levi Montalcini 1952; Calissano et al. 1984). It exerts a crucial role in the survival and differentiation of neural crest-derived cells such as sensory, sympathetic and chromaffin cells. However, NGF deprivation during fetal life results not only in a dramatic degeneration of these cells in the neonates, but also in a complex neuroendocrine deficiency (Aloe et al. 1981; Johnson et al. 1980). This led to the suggestion that the action of NGF may be broader than at first envisaged. Furthermore, it has been recently shown that NGF might also promote the growth and the differentiation of mast cells (Aloe and Levi Montalcini 1977). Prompted by such observations and by a more general interest in the relatedness between the nervous and the immune system, I investigated the possibility that new target cells for NGF hitherto unrecognized may be found among lymphoid cells. The results, which will be presented below, show that a well-defined subset of rat thymocytes possess membrane receptors for NGF and allow one to postulate that NGF may play a role in the maturation and/or differentiation of such cells.

The presence of NGF membrane receptors was assessed on cell suspensions from bone marrow, spleen and thymus of two-month-old rats. Whereas bone marrow or spleen cells do not display any specific binding of NGF, thymocytes do show a specific NGF binding (Fig. 1), whose affinity is 1.5×10^{-9} M, a value which is very close to the affinity of the NGF receptors on PC12 cells (Fig. 1). The NGF-binding capacity of thymocytes is very low, if calculated on a total cell basis (200–800 NGF molecules/cell as compared to $5-7 \times 10^4$ NGF molecules/PC12 cell) (Fig. 1). The low binding capacity can be due either to a low number of receptors on all thymus cells, or to the binding of NGF to a subset of the total cells. Due to the cellular and functional heterogeneity of the thymus, the second possibility is more likely, and indeed, different lines of evidence demonstrate that NGF binds only to a subpopulation of thymocytes and lead to a first identification of such cells. Different monoclonal antibodies to rat membrane antigens have been described (Mason et al. 1983). These antibodies allow four distinct subpopulations to be defined in the rat thymus, corresponding to different maturation stages and/or lineages, and they have been used in the present study in the attempt of characterizing the cells within the thymus bearing

1   Istituto di Biologia Cellulare C.N.R., Roma, Italy

Molecular Aspects of Neurobiology
(ed. by Rita Levi Montalcini et al.)
© Springer Verlag Berlin Heidelberg 1986

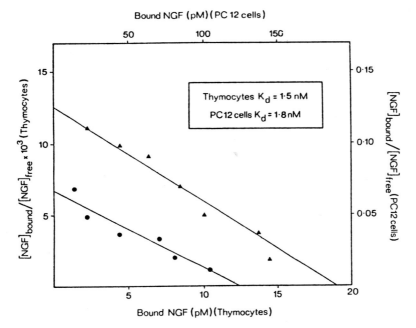

Fig. 1. ^{125}I-NGF binding to rat thymocytes (▲) and PC12 cells (●). Specific binding is reported as a Scatchard plot. The binding refers to 0.5×10^6 PC12 cells/point and to 20×10^6 thymocytes/point

NGF receptors. Firstly, the binding of ^{125}I-NGF to thymocytes was measured after a treatment which leads to selective survival of medullary thymocytes. Culturing thymocytes for 3 days with Concanavalin A or with Phytohaemoagglutinin plus ConA-activated spleen cells supernatant yields a 100% recovery of the NGF binding capacity. Moreover, since such a treatment causes the selective loss of cortical thymocytes (representing approximately 80% of total thymocytes) the NGF-binding capacity expressed on a per cell basis increases from 0.2 fmoles bound NGF/10^6 cells (freshly dissociated thymocytes) to 1.2 fmoles bound NGF/10^6 cells (thymocytes cultured with lectins) (see Table 1). The cell surface phenotype of the cells before and after incubation with lectins was determined by flow cytofluorimetry, using the panel of monoclonal antibodies mentioned above. The surface labeling pattern of lectin-treated thymocytes (Table 1) is in keeping with the notion that this cell population results from the selective survival and expansion of a functionally mature subpopulation within the thymus, cortical immature cells dying readily both in culture conditions and in vivo. This is particularly evident if the labeling by the NR5/10 antibody (which recognizes the rat Class I Major Histocompatibility Complex antigen) is considered: while around 15% of the untreated thymocytes are labeled by this antibody, this figure increases to 90% after lectin stimulation (Table 1). Therefore, it may be concluded that the selective loss of cortical thymocytes (which do not express the Class I MHC antigen) with this culture condition does not affect the NGF binding capacity of the overall thymocyte subpopulation. In order to answer the question whether the

Table 1. Binding of NGF and surface phenotype of thymocytes cultures with lectins.
Thymocytes were cultured at a concentration of 2×10^6/ml for 3 days, in the presence of 1%
Phytohaemoagglutinin (PHA) and 20% of a supernatant from Con A stimulated rat spleen cells.
Cells were cultured in the presence or in the absence of 100 ng/ml NGF. At the end of the incubation aliquots of the cells were incubated with the antibodies and staining was revealed by analysis
on a fluorescence activated cell sorter (FACS II). Binding of NGF was measured as described. A
suspension of fresh thymocytes was analyzed in parallel. NGF binding is expressed as fmoles/10^6
cells

Cells	NGF binding	OX7	OX8	OX19	W3/25	NR5/10
Fresh thymocytes	0.2	69%$^{2+}$ 26%$^+$	70%	10%$^{2+}$ 89%$^+$	78%	15%
PHA	1.2	25%$^{2+}$ 31%$^+$	73%	36%$^{2+}$ 62%$^+$	42%	90%
PHA + NGF	n.t.	17%$^{2+}$ 31%$^+$	80%	60%$^{2+}$ 40%$^+$	53%	90%

NGF receptors on thymocytes are functional, the effect of NGF on the surface phenotype of the lectin-stimulated thymocytes was also determined (Table 1). The results
of such an analysis demonstrate that while the percentage of thymocytes labeled by
the antibodies MRC OX-7, MRC OX-8 and W3/25 is slightly but significantly modified
by culturing thymocytes with NGF, the MRC OX-19 bright (OX19^{2+}) cells increase
from 34% in the absence of NGF to 60% after incubation with the factor (Table 1).
The number of cells expressing the Class I MHC antigen does not vary upon incubation
with NGF (note that 90% of the lectin stimulated thymocytes express such a marker),
but the distribution shifts to higher staining intensity: 54% of the cells are found at
fluorescence intensities greater than channel 80 in control cultures and 65.5% in NGF
treated cultures. Such effect is not due to an increase in the cell size, as measured by
light scattering (not shown). These findings, together with the observation that incubation of thymocytes with NGF for 3 days leads to a 70% reduction of their lectin-
induced ^{3}H-thymidine incorporation (Cattaneo and Secher, submitted), shows that the
binding of NGF to its receptors on thymocytes mediates measurable effects, thus
demonstrating that these receptors can be functional. It cannot be concluded at the
present stage whether the effects described reflect a direct action of NGF on the cells
bearing receptors or whether they result from an indirect interaction occurring within
the heterogeneous cell population.

Mature, medullary-type thymocytes appear, from the experiment reported above,
to possess receptors for NGF. Such cells, while having a number of similar membrane
markers (e.g. Class I MHC antigen) can be further subdivided with the antibodies
W3/25, which labels medullary cells of the T helper lineage, and MRC OX-8, which
labels cells of the suppressor-cytotoxic lineage. Both antibodies also label the bulk of
cortical immature thymocytes. Complement killing experiments have been performed
with these antibodies. The result of the experiment with antibody W3/25, which labels
94% of thymocytes (see inset of Fig. 2), is shown in Fig. 2 and demonstrates that the
binding of NGF was unaffected by the killing of over 90% of the thymocytes with

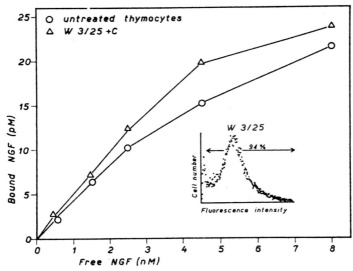

Fig. 2. ^{125}I-NGF binding to thymocytes treated with antibody W3/25 and complement. The inset shows the fluorescence labeling intensity profile of thymocytes after incubation with antibody W3/25. The treatment with complement killed 90.5% of the cells. Nonspecific killing, measured with a nonrelevant antibody, was less than 4%

W3/25 plus complement. Therefore, NGF receptor bearing cells are not contained among the W3/25[+] cells. Further complement killing experiments demonstrate that whereas killing of the thymocytes expressing high levels of the Thy 1 antigen (supposedly immature, cortical thymocytes) does not affect NGF binding, killing of the thymocytes expressing the Class I MHC antigen reduces the binding of NGF by 65% (Cattaneo and Secher, submitted). From these experiments it may be concluded that a small subset of thymocytes displays NGF receptors. These cells express the Class I MHC antigen, the OX-8 antigen, low levels of Thy 1 and are W3/25[−]. As mentioned above, the OX-8 antigen distinguishes thymocytes of the T suppressor and cytotoxic lineage. Moreover, a distinct type of T lymphocyte (derived from the thymus) recently described, the gut intramucosal T lymphocyte, is OX-8[+] (Lyscom and Brueton 1982). This cell type has been proposed to give rise to the so called "atypical" mucosal mast cells, a subset of mast cells for which the arguments for an origin from the thymus are most compelling, although not conclusive (Burnet 1977). In view of the evidence relating NGF to mast cells (Aloe and Levi Montalcini 1977; Bruni et al. 1982) it is tempting to speculate that the subset of thymocytes with NGF receptors contains the precursors of the gut T lymphocyte and/or of mucosal mast cells. Thus, NGF may act on both type of mast cells, or mast cell precursors, the connective tissue mast cells (e.g. peritoneal mast cells) and the "atypical" mucosal mast cells. Given the bone marrow origin of the first type of mast cells, the subset of thymocytes described in the present paper could possibly relate to the second type of mast cells, in view of the presence of the OX-8 marker on the NGF bearing thymocytes. On the other hand, the possibility of a role of NGF on the connective tissue mast cells is strengthened by the

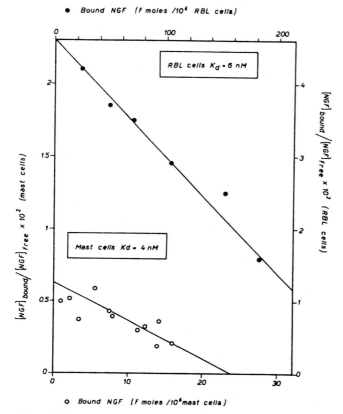

Fig. 3. ^{125}I-NGF binding to rat peritoneal mast cells (o) and to a rat basophilic leukemia cell line (RBL cells) (•)

observation that also peritoneal mast cells display receptors for NGF, although of lower affinity than those on PC12 cells or on thymocytes (see Fig. 3). Interestingly, also a subclone of rat basophilic leukemia cells (RBL cells), which is the clonal cell line most widely used as a model for mast cells and IgE-mediated release of histamine, displays NGF receptors, in the number of 3×10^4/cell (see Fig. 3). This clonal cell line may prove in the future to be a valuable model system to study the interactions between NGF and these non-neuronal target cells.

The results presented may represent another facet of the connections between the nervous and the immune system. We are now in the position, moreover, of critically testing the hypothesis that a well defined subset of cells in the thymus may be dependent on NGF for its maturation, utilizing the experimental approach of immunological deprivation of endogenous NGF which has been so important for the demonstration of the role of NGF in neuronal differentiation (Levi Montalcini 1966).

Acknowledgments. I wish to express my gratitude to P. Calissano and R. Levi Montalcini for helpful discussion. I am also greatly indebted to D.S. Secher (MRC Laboratory of Molecular Biology, Cambridge U.K.) in whose laboratory part of this work was performed. Part of this work has been supported by a grant Progetto Finalizzato Oncologia del C.N.R. to P. Calissano.

References

Aloe L, Levi Montalcini R (1977) Mast cells increase in tissues of neonatal rats injected with the nerve growth factor. Brain Res 133:358–366

Aloe L, Cozzari C, Calissano P, Levi Montalcini R (1981) Somatic and behavioural postnatal effects of fetal injections of nerve growth factor antibodies in the rat. Nature 291:413–415

Bruni A, Bigon E, Boarato E, Mietto L, Leon A, Toffano G (1982) Interaction between nerve growth factor and lysophosphatidylserine on rat peritoneal mast cells. FEBS Lett 138:190–192

Burnet (1977) The probable relationship of some or all mast cells to the T-cell system. Cell Immunol 30:358–360

Calissano P, Cattaneo A, Aloe L, Levi Montalcini R (1984) The nerve growth factor (NGF). In: Li CH (ed) Hormonal proteins and peptides. Growth factors. Academic, New York, p 1

Johnson EM, Gorin PD, Brandeis LD, Pearson J (1980) Dorsal root ganglion neurons are destroyed by exposure in utero to maternal antibody to nerve growth factor. Science 210:916–918

Levi Montalcini R (1952) Effects of mouse tumor transplantation on the nervous system. Ann NY Acad Sci 55:330–343

Levi Montalcini R (1966) The nerve growth factor: its mode of action on sensory and sympathetic nerve cells. Harvey Lect 60:217–259

Lyscom N, Brueton MJ (1982) Intraepithelial, lamina propria and Peyer's patch lymphocytes of the rat small intestine: isolation and characterization in terms of immunoglobulin markers and receptors for monoclonal antibodies. Immunology 45:775–783

Mason DW, Arthur RP, Dallman RJ, Green JR, Spickett GP, Thomas ML (1983) Functions of rat T lymphocyte subsets isolated by means of monoclonal antibodies. Immunol Rev 74:57–82

Expression of the *v-src* Oncogene Induces Differentiation in PC12 Cells

P. CASALBORE[1], E. AGOSTINI[1], F. TATÒ[2], and S. ALEMÀ[1]

PC12 rat pheochromocytoma cells respond to nerve growth factor (NGF) protein (Calissano et al. 1984) by acquiring a new phenotype characterized by emission of neurites and increased expression of sympathetic neuron functions (Greene and Tischler 1982). In spite of extensive efforts, however, the intracellular events that in PC12 cells transduce the signals from recepetor-bound NGF remain largely elusive. It is an established finding that expression of viral oncogenes in cells belonging to different lineages is accompanied by a specific derangement in the synthesis of differentiated products (Holtzer et al. 1982; Falcone et al. 1985). In this report we present data on the effect of infection of PC12 cells with retroviruses carrying the *src* oncogene of Rous sarcoma virus (RSV) (Weiss et al. 1982).

PC12 cells were infected with the mammaltropic strain Schmidt Ruppin D (SR-D) of RSV and other mammaltropic viral strains and their conditional mutants (Weiss et al. 1982). After a lag of about 48–72 h after infection, a variable proportion (up to 20%, depending on m.o.i. and experiment) of cells started to undergo a marked phenotypic conversion as shown by the emission of short and long neurites. PC12 cells infected with the temperature-sensitive (ts) mutant LA339-B77, and passaged at 39°C were indistinguishable from uninfected controls. Following a shift to 35°C, however, the ts-LA339-infected cells differentiated within 2–3 days, thus suggesting that differentiation required a functional pp60^{v-src}, the *src* gene product (Weiss et al. 1982). Transformation-defective mutants of B77 and non-mammaltropic strains were ineffective. Antibodies directed against NGF did not inhibit the outgrowth elicited by RSV infection. No neurite extension was detected when tissue culture fluids from SR-D-infected PC12 cultures were tested for induction of morphological differentiation in uninfected cells.

SR-D-infected and differentiated cells remain viable when cultivated in serum-free conditions, whereas undifferentiated ones die within a few days. This property has been exploited as a simple means to obtain cultures highly enriched in differentiated cells (Fig. 1) suitable for assaying the expression of constitutive (storage of catecholamines and α-bungarotoxin binding sites) and differentiation-induced (AChE and neurofilament proteins) markers of the PC12 cell line. Both former markers were not

1   Istituto di Biologia Cellulare, C.N.R., Via G. Romagnosi 18/A, Roma, Italy
2   Dipartimento di Biologia Cellulare e dello Sviluppo, Università di Roma "La Sapienza", Roma, Italy

Molecular Aspects of Neurobiology
(ed. by Rita Levi Montalcini et al.)
© Springer-Verlag Berlin Heidelberg 1986

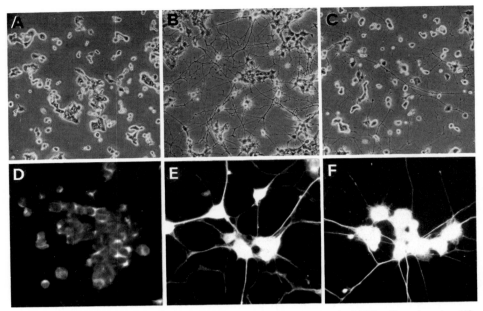

Fig. 1A–F. Neurite extension and neurofilament protein expression in PC12 cells undergoing differentiation. Phase-contrast (A–C) and immunofluorescence (D–F) of control uninfected PC12 cells (A,D), NGF-treated cells (B,E) and SR-D-infected cells, enriched through serum deprivation (C,F)

significantly altered in SR-D-infected cultures, while the same cultures expressed increased (threefold) levels of AChE and increased synthesis and assembly of neurofilament proteins (Fig. 1D–F). Next we asked whether these differentiated cells could synthesize DNA or whether differentiation is accompanied by a progressive withdrawal from the cell cycle, as shown previously for NGF-treated PC12 cells (Greene and Tischler 1982). Autoradiographic studies showed that while the vast majority of control PC12 cells, grown in serum, were labeled, a fraction of serum-free enriched, highly differentiated cells had ceased to incorporate tritiated thymidine. To further substantiate that the emission of neurites was under the control of the *src* gene, we tested the presence of pp60$^{v\text{-}src}$ in RSV-infected cultures using the immune complex kinase assay (Collett and Erikson 1978). SR-D-infected PC12 cells at 7 days post-infection contained elevated levels of pp60$^{v\text{-}src}$, comparable to those of a SR-D transformed clone of the rat myogenic cell line L8 (Fig. 2A). Differentiated, serum-free enriched cells showed a threefold increase in kinase activity, a finding strongly indicating that differentiated cells express levels of kinase usually associated with transformation in other rat cell types. Levels of pp60$^{c\text{-}src}$, the cellular *src*-kinase activity (Weiss et al. 1982) remained constant when assayed 10 days after addition of NGF or infection by RSV (Fig. 2B).

Contrary to other cellular systems, where the effect of *src* appears to involve a direct and specific suppression of a given differentiation program (Holtzer et al. 1982; Falcone et al. 1985), in PC12 cells expression of *v-src* has an inductive effect

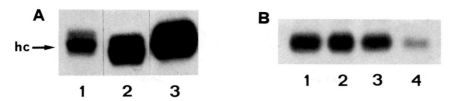

Fig. 2A,B. Expression of pp60^{src} in uninfected and RSV-infected PC12 cells. the *src* kinase activity capable of phosphorylating the heavy chain of IgG (hc) was measured as described in Collett and Erikson (1978). **A** pp60$^{v\text{-}src}$ activity in cell extracts of SR-D-infected PC12 cells before (*1*) or after (*2*) selection through serum deprivation and clonal SR-D-transformed L8 cells (*3*). **B** pp60$^{c\text{-}src}$ activity in extracts of control uninfected (*1*), NGF-treated (*2*), SR-D-infected (*3*) PC12 cells and uninfected Rat-1 cells (*4*)

on differentiation that closely resembles that of NGF. The present findings suggest a possible relationship between the mechanism of action of NGF and the biochemical events that are associated with *src*-induced transformation, such as tyrosine phosphorylation of proteins (Weiss et al. 1982) or increased turnover of the phosphoinositides (Majerus et al. 1984). In particular it remains to be assessed whether *v-src* triggers an aberrant type of differentiation in PC12 cells or whether it shares with NGF a common pathway.

Acknowledgment. Supported by a CNR-PF Medicina Preventiva grant.

References

Calissano P, Cattaneo A, Aloe L, Levi Montalcini R (1984) The nerve growth factor (NGF). In: Li CH (ed) Hormonal proteins and peptides. Academic, New York, pp 1–56

Collett MS, Erikson RL (1978) Protein kinase activity associated with the avian sarcoma virus *src* gene product. Proc Natl Acad Sci USA 75:2021–2024

Falcone G, Tatò F, Alemà S (1985) Distinctive effects of the viral oncogenes *myc, erb, fps* and *src* on the differentiation program of quail myogenic cells. Proc Natl Acad Sci USA 82:426–430

Greene LA, Tischler AS (1982) Adv Cell Neurobiol 3:373–414

Holtzer H, Pacifici M, Tapscott S, Bennett G, Payette R, Dlugosz A (1982) Lineages in cell differentiation and in cell transformation. In: Revoltella et al. (eds) Expression of differentiated functions in tumour cells. Raven, New York, pp 169–180

Majerus PW, Neufeld EJ, Wilson DB (1984) Production of phosphoinositide-derived messengers. Cell 37:701–703

Weiss RA, Teich NM, Varmus HE, Coffin JM (eds) (1982) RNA tumour viruses. Cold Spring Harbour Laboratory, Cold Spring Harbour, NY

Serum Influences β-NGF Gene Expression in Mouse L Cells

R. HOULGATTE, D. WION, P. BARRAND, E. DICOU, and P. BRACHET[1]

L-929 cells derive from a mouse connective tissue (Earle 1943). They secrete a neuro-trophic factor which is immunologically and biochemically similar to the β-NGF found in mouse submaxillary glands (Oger et al. 1974; Brachet and Dicou 1984). Hybridiza-tions with a β-NGF cDNA probe (Scott et al. 1983) have recently shown that L cells contain a β-NGF transcript identical in size to that produced by the submaxillary gland, and that the β-NGF locus of the genomic DNA is not rearranged, as evidenced by cleavage with some restriction enzymes (Wion et al. 1985). L cells, therefore, constitute a valuable model system suited for the study of the gene expression of the factor. The present work deals with a preliminary characterization of extracellular effector molecules which influence this expression. Extracellular concentrations of β-NGF were correlated with intracellular levels of the β-NGF mRNA in cells cultured in the presence or absence of serum, or exposed to testosterone, T3 or T4, which are known to enhance the β-NGF levels in the mouse submaxillary gland (Levi Montalcini and Angeletti 1968; Aloe and Levi Montalcini 1980).

Methods

Assay of β-NGF. L cells were grown in serum-free medium (Darmon et al. 1982) dur-ing 2 days before they were supplemented with the compounds indicated in Table 1. After 24 h, the factor was measured in the supernatants with the double site ELISA assay described by Furukawa et al. (1983), except that we used Dynatech microelisa plates and a mouse monoclonal anti-β-NGF antibody (Korsching and Thoenen 1983). Recoveries were verified by adding a known amount of pure β-NGF in part of the samples. Other samples were incubated with an excess of anti-β-NGF immunoglobulins before the enzyme-linked antibodies were added in order to obtain background values. The limit of sensibility ranged between $2-10$ pg β-NGF/ml.

Total RNA was extracted from L cells and samples containing identical amounts of polyadenylated RNA, previously quantified by hybridization with (^{3}H)poly(U), were subjected to dot blot analysis by hybridization with the (^{32}P)-labeled β-NGF cDNA

---

1 Unité de Différenciation Cellulaire, Institut Pasteur, 25 rue du Dr. Roux, Paris Cedex 15, France

Molecular Aspects of Neurobiology
(ed. by Rita Levi Montalcini et al.)
© Springer-Verlag Berlin Heidelberg 1986

Table 1. Extracellular levels of β-NGF and intracellular levels of its mRNA

Culture conditions	β-NGF ng/10^7 cells/24 h ± SEM (n)		β-NGF-RNA (relative amounts) ± SEM (n)	
5% horse serum	33.2 ± 5.6	(5)	100	
Serum-free	5.5 ± 0.17	(5)	23.7 ± 4.3	(6)
+ Testosterone 10^{-7} M	4.7 ± 0.66	(5)	22 ± 2.3	(3)
+ T3 10^{-7} M	9.81 ± 2.6	(5)	38 ± 4	(4)
+ T4 10^{-7} M	9.7 ± 2.0	(5)	35.5	(1)

(Thomas 1980). Relative amounts of β-NGF mRNA were estimated by densitometric scanning of the radioautograms, and further verified by northern blot analysis of agarose gels. A value of 100 was attributed to the relative amounts found in cells cultured with serum. The complete experimental procedure is described in details elsewhere (Wion et al. 1985).

Results

As shown in Table 1, the biosynthesis of β-NGF by L cells can be modulated by the culture conditions. The close relationship between intracellular β-NGF mRNA concentrations and the amounts of the extracellular factor indicates that the regulatory mechanism probably operates at some pretranslational level. Highest levels of β-NGF mRNAs and of secreted factor were observed in cells cultured with serum. This suggests that some seric factor(s) induces the transcription of the β-NGF gene or stabilizes its transcript. The β-NGF mRNA levels were also increased when cells were grown in serum-free medium supplemented with T3 or T4. In contrast, testosterone had no effect.

In order to characterize further the seric factor which influences the levels of β-NGF transcripts, the serum was dialyzed, or heated for 15 min at 50° or 60°C, or treated with Dowex AG1-X8, which is known to remove most of the thyroid hormones T3 or T4 (Samuels et al. 1979). Measurements of the extracellular β-NGF concentrations in L cells cultured for 24 h with such treated sera are reported in Table 2.

Table 2. Secretion of β-NGF by L cells ng/10^7 cells/24 h ± SEM (n)

Treatment of serum No.	Dialyzed	AG1-X8	50°C	60°C
33.2 ± 5.6	33.1 ± 5.3	33.1 ± 4.9	31.9 ± 6.0	13.0 ± 2.1
(5)	(4)	(4)	(3)	(4)

Clearly, the stimulation exerted by the serum is not due to endogenous T3 or T4 hormones since treatment with Dowex AG1-X8 did not alter its effect. It should be stressed that seric concentrations of free T3 or T4 are much lower than those quoted in Table 1. The seric effector behaves as a high molecular weight molecule, for it was not removed by dialysis. It appears thermolabile, since its activity declined significantly after mild heat treatment.

Several reports have shown that the production of β-NGF by peripheral tissues can be significantly enhanced when they are transplanted in vitro, and cultured in presence of serum (Ebendal et al. 1980; Harper et al. 1980; Shelton and Reichardt 1984). Our data raise the possibility that this induction is in part mediated by the seric effector active on L cells.

References

Aloe L, Levi Montalcini R (1980) Comparative studies on testosterone and L-thyroxine effects on the synthesis of NGF in the mouse submaxillary salivary glands. Exp Cell Res 125:15–22

Brachet P, Dicou E (1984) L-cells potentiate the effect of the extracellular NGF activity in co-cultures with PC12 pheochromocytoma cells. Exp Cell Res 150:234–241

Darmon M, Buc-Caron MH, Paulin D, Jacob F (1982) Control by the extracellular environment of differentiation pathways in 1003 embryonal carcinoma cells. EMBO J 1:901–906

Earle WR (1943) Production of malignancy in vitro. The mouse fibroblast cultures and changes seen in the living cells. J Natl Cancer Inst 4:165–212

Ebendal T, Olson L, Seiger A, Hedlung KO (1980) Nerve growth factors in the rat iris. Nature 286: 25–28

Furukawa S, Kamo I, Furukawa Y, Akazawa S, Satoyoshi F, Itok K, Kayashi K (1983) A highly sensitive enzyme immunoassay for mouse β-NGF. J Neurochem 40:734–743

Harper GP, Al-Saffar A, Pearce F, Vernon C (1980) The production of NGF in vitro by tissues of mouse, rat and embryonic chick. Dev Biol 77:379–390

Korsching S, Thoenen H (1983) NGF in sympathetic ganglia and corresponding target organs of the rat: correlation with density of sympathetic innervation. Proc Natl Acad Sci USA 80: 3513–3516

Levi Montalcini R, Angeletti PU (1968) Nerve growth factor. Physiol Rev 48:534–569

Oger J, Arnason B, Pantazis N, Lehrich J, Young M (1974) Synthesis of NGF by L and 3T3 cells in culture. Proc Natl Acad Sci USA 71:1554–1558

Samuels HH, Stanley F, Casanova J (1979) Depletion of L-(3,5,3') tri-iodothyronine and L-thyroxine in euthyroid calf serum for use in cell culture studies of the action of thyroid hormone. Endocrinology 105:80–85

Scott J, Selby M, Urdea M, Quiroga M, Bell G, Rutter W (1983) Isolation and nucleotide sequence of a cDNA encoding the precursor of mouse NGF. Nature 302:538–540

Shelton P, Reichardt L (1984) Expression of the β-NGF gene correlates with the density of sympathetic innervation in effector organs. Proc Natl Acad Sci USA 81:7951–7955

Thomas P (1980) Hybridisation of denatured DNA and small DNA fragments transferred to nitrocellulose. Proc Natl Acad Sci USA 77:5201–5205

Wion D, Barrand P, Dicou E, Brachet P (1985) Serum and thyroid hormones T3 and T4 regulate NGF mRNA levels in mouse L cells. FEBS Lett 189:37–41

Isolation of Glia Maturation Factor with HPLC and Verification with a Monoclonal Antibody

R. LIM and J.F. MILLER[1]

1. Introduction

Glia maturation factor (GMF), discovered in our laboratory (Lim et al. 1972, 1973; Lim and Mitsunobu 1974), is one of the first brain-derived growth factors reported (Lim 1980, 1985). These factors often have target cells within the nervous system and thus may have autoregulatory functions in brain development, repair and regeneration. GMF is an acidic protein extractable at neutral pH from the mature brain of various species. In addition to promoting the proliferation and differentiation of astrocytes, GMF is also a mitogen for Schwann cells. GMF stimulates astrocytes to produced second order hormones such as interleukin-1 and prostaglandins. When added to cultures of glial tumor cells, GMF partially reverses the malignant process by promoting contact inhibition. The isolation of this biologically active protein is essential to the understanding of its mechanism of action.

2. Purification of GMF with Reverse Phase HPLC

We previously partially purified GMF from bovine brains by the following steps: ammonium sulfate precipitation, DEAE Sephacel column, Sephadex G-75 column and hydroxylapatite column (Lim and Miller 1984). We now have proceeded one step further by using high performance liquid chromatography (HPLC), obtaining a product with apparent homogeneity. Forty ml of the GFM sample eluted from the hydroxyl-apatite column was dialyzed against 0.1 M ammonium formate and lyophilized. The material was taken up in 2 ml of 20% acetonitrile (AN) containing 0.1% trifluoroacetic acid (TFA) and loaded on a 4.6 mm × 5 cm C4 Vydac HPLC column. The charged column was washed with 20 ml of the same solvent mixture and eluted with 40 ml of a linear gradient of 20–45% acetonitrile containing 0.1% TFA, at a flow rate of 1.5 ml/min. The GMF activity peak emerged between 35% and 40% acetonitrile concentration. This fraction was collected, and similar fractions from three parallel runs were pooled and rechromatographed with the same HPLC column under identical

1 Veterans Administration Medical Center and Department of Neurology
   (Division of Neurochemistry and Neurobiology), University of Iowa, Iowa City, IA 52242, USA

Molecular Aspects of Neurobiology
(ed. by Rita Levi Montalcini et al.)
© Springer-Verlag Berlin Heidelberg 1986

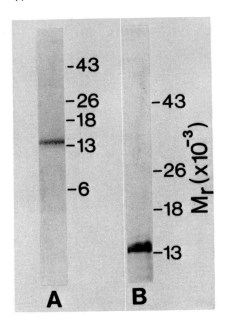

Fig. 1A,B. SDS polyacrylamide gel electrophoresis (PAGE) of purified GMF under reducing conditions. **A** 10 ng GMF in 18% gel. **B** 100 ng GMF in 12% gel. Silver stained

conditions. The elution profile showed a single protein peak (absorbance at 214 nm) coinciding with the activity peak at the expected acetonitrile concentration, resulting in a 100,000-fold overall purification starting from the crude brain extract.

The final product showed a single protein band, with a molecular weight of 14,000, on SDS polyacrylamide gel electrophoresis under reducing conditions (Fig. 1). Electrofocusing on LKB plates revealed an isoelectric point of pH 5.2. When assayed with rat astroblasts, the purified GMF exhibited both mitogenic (thymidine incorporation) and morphogenic (cell process outgrowth) effects as with the cruder preparations, with maximum activity at 40 ng/ml and half maximum activity at 8 ng/ml (Fig. 2).

3. Production of Monoclonal Antibody and Immunological Verification

Female Balb/c mice, 8-weeks-old, were immunized with GMF through four injections, each consisted of 750 μg of partially purified GMF obtained through the hydroxylapatite step. The first injection was given subcutaneously with complete Freund's adjuvant, and the subsequent injections were given intraperitoneally with incomplete Freund's adjuvant. After verifying the response with tail bleed, the spleen cells were fused with the NS1 myeloma cell line and the resulting hybridomas were screened for the production of antibodies against GMF. This was carried out with the ELISA procedure, using β-galactosidase as the indicator system, first against partially purified GMF, then against pure GMF.

One of the positive clones, designated as G2-09, was extensively characterized. Adsorption with the antibody (IgG_{2b}) led to the inactivation of GMF activity, both

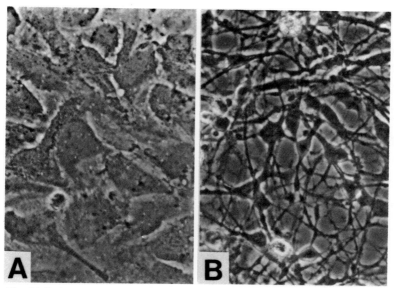

Fig. 2A,B. Morphological effect of purified GMF in confluent cultures of rat astroblasts in the presence of 5% fetal calf serum. A Cells not exposed to GMF. B Cells exposed to GMF for 2 days at 40 ng/ml

mitogenic and morphogenic, in a dose related manner (Fig. 3). In order to show that this antibody indeed was directed toward the GMF protein, GMF samples were electro-phoresed on SDS gels and electroblotted on nitrocellulose sheets followed by incuba-tion with the antibody. The monoclonal antibody consistently identified the 14,000 kd protein band as the antigen, both in pure and in partially purified GMF (Fig. 4). Immunoblotting of an isoelectrically focused GMF sample yielded similar results. Thus, the monoclonal antibody relates the biological activity to the putative GMF protein band, establishing the identity of the purified protein as GMF.

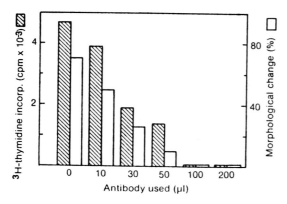

Fig. 3. Adsorption of GMF activity (mitogenic and morphogenic) by monoclonal antibody. The assay was conducted on rat astroblasts

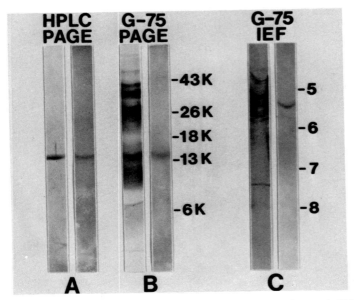

Fig. 4A–C. Immunoblotting of GMF by monoclonal antibody. A HPLC-purified GMF in SDS-PAGE. B Sephadex G-75 partially purified GMF in SDS-PAGE. C Sephadex G-75 partially purified GMF after isoelectric focusing. Gels are on the *left*; immunoblots on the *right*. Molecular weights are indicated for SDS gels; pH values are indicated for IEF gel

4. Discussion

Although GMF was discovered over a decade ago, past attempts to purify GMF resulted in only partial success, mainly due to the instability of the protein when it was close to purity. Thanks to HPLC which effectively resolves GMF from its last contaminants under conditions that do not denature GMF, we have now purified GMF to apparent homogeneity. The success in purification is indeed a major advance in GMF research, as the availability of pure GMF is a prerequisite to the meaningful study of its molecular structure and mechanism of action.

Growth factors are regulatory molecules that control the proliferation and/or maturation of various cell types. Attention has recently been focused on the relatedness of some growth factors or their receptors to the oncogenes. Several of the growth factors have similar though not identical chemical and biological properties, indicating a possibly common evolutionary origin. The isolation and identification of the individual factors, including GMF, provides essential groundwork for a systematic comparison of these biologically important molecules.

5. Summary

Bovine glia maturation factor (GMF) has been purified 100,000-fold through multiple steps including a final step with reverse phase HPLC. A monoclonal antibody raised against partially purified GMF adsorbs GMF activity and identifies the putative GMF protein band as the antigen.

Acknowledgments. Supported by the following grants to Dr. Lim: VA Merit Review and Career Investigatorship Awards, NSF grant BNS-8308341, NCI grant CA-31796, Diabetes-Endocrinology Research Center Grant AM-25295, and University of Iowa Cancer Center Grant.

References

Lim R (1980) Glia maturation factor. In: Moscona AA, Monroy A, Hunt RK (eds) Current topics in developmental biology, vol 16. Academic, New York, p 305

Lim R (1985) Glia maturation factor and other factors acting on glia. In: Guroff G (ed) Growth and maturation factors, vol 3. John Wiley, New York, p 119

Lim R, Miller JF (1984) An improved procedure for the isolation of glia maturation factor. J Cell Physiol 119:255–259

Lim R, Mitsunobu K (1974) Brain cells in culture: morphological transformation by a protein. Science 185:63–66

Lim R, Li WKP, Mitsunobu K (1972) Morphological transformation of dissociated embryonic brain cells in the presence of brain extracts. Abstr 2nd Annu Meet Soc Neurosci, Houston, TX, p 181

Lim R, Mitsunobu K, Li WKP (1973) Maturation-stimulating effect of brain extract and dibutyryl cyclic AMP on dissociated embryonic brain cells in culture. Exp Cell Res 79:243–246

Nicotinic Receptors from Different Peripheral Organs and from Brain are Highly Homologous, Complex Proteins

B.M. CONTI-TRONCONI[1], M.A. RAFTERY[2], and S.M.J. DUNN[2]

1. Torpedo Acetylcholine Receptor

The acetylcholine receptor (AChR) from *Torpedo* electroplax can be isolated in a pure form either in its native membrane-bound state or by affinity chromatography after solubilization. Due to the ease with which this receptor can be purified, both its structure and its function have been investigated to a remarkable degree of sophistication.

It is now established that *Torpedo* AChR is formed by four different proteins which in *T. californica* have, upon SDS gel electrophoresis, apparent molecular weights of 40,000, 50,000, 60,000 and 65,000, commonly referred to as α, β, γ and δ, respectively (see Conti-Tronconi and Raftery 1982). This complex structure was challenged for many years by reports of pure AChR having simpler subunit patterns but these erroneous reports are now known to have been the result of proteolytic artifacts (reviewed in Conti-Tronconi and Raftery 1982). The subunit pattern of *Torpedo* AChR is very sensitive to proteolysis, and it can be cleaved or nicked to the extent that only the α chain retains its integrity, without significant effect on the functional and structural characteristics of AChR.

The debate regarding the subunit composition of AChR was resolved by the demonstration that the four peptides present in pure AChR preparations are highly homologous proteins (Raftery et al. 1980; Fig. 1). It was further demonstrated directly by simultaneous quantitative sequencing of the mixture of polypeptides obtained by SDS denaturation of purified, intact AChR that the four subunits are present in the AChR molecule with a stoichiometry of $\alpha_2\beta\gamma\delta$, in excellent agreement with the value determined previously for the M_r of the complex (Martinez-Carrion et al. 1975).

In the recent past, the complete amino acid sequence of the precursors of all *Torpedo* subunits has been deduced from corresponding nucleic acid clones obtained by recombinant DNA technology. This has shown that the subunits have homologous sequences throughout their length (Noda et al. 1983). The extensive homology of the four AChR subunits argues for a shared ancestry and allows the generation of a pseudosymmetric complex similar to that observed for many complex proteins (Raftery et al. 1980).

1 Department of Biochemistry, University of Minnesota, St. Paul, MN 55108, USA
2 The Braun Laboratories of the Division of Chemistry, California Institute of Technology, Pasadena, CA 91125, USA

Molecular Aspects of Neurobiology
(ed. by Rita levi Montalcini et al.)
© Springer-Verlag Berlin Heidelberg 1986

Torpedo AChR

alpha	SEHETRLVANLL	ENYNKVIRPVEHHTHFVDITVGLQLIQLISVDEVNQIVETNV
beta	SVMEDTLLSVLF	ETYNPKVRPAQTVGDKVTVRVGLTLTNLLILNEKIEEMRTNV
gamma	ENEEGRLIEKLL	GDYDKRIIPAKTLDHIIDVTLKLTLTNLISLNEMEEALTTNV
delta	VNEEERLINDLLLIVNKYNKHVRPVKHNNEVVNIALSLTLSNLISLKETDETLTSNV

conserved * * *   *   *   * * *   *   **

Electrophorus

alpha	SEDETRLVKNLF	SGYNKVVRPVNH
beta	SEAENDLMNKLF	TAYNPKVRPAEK
gamma	NEESDLIADKF	TNYNKLIRPAKH
delta	RNEEERLINHLFKERGYNKELRPAQT

conserved * * *   * *

Fetal Calf

alpha   SEHETRLVAKLF   EDYNPVVRPVEDH?DAVVVNVGL

beta   SEAEERLNEKLF   SEYNP^V_KV^F_EPA^E_PTVR

x   ?EHENKLQAHLF   DDYAS$^{HK}_{KP}$FP?^E_R

y   ?NEEE^R_NLL$^?_R$DLF$^{?E}_{FL}$KAYNK^E_FL?PA

conserved   * *   **   *   *

Alpha Subunits

chick muscle	✗EHETRLVDDLFRDYSKVVRPVENH
chick brain	✗EFETKLYKELLKNYNPLE?PVA?D
fetal calf	SEHETRLVAKLFEDYNSVVRPVEDH
Torpedo	SEHETRLVANLLENYNKVIRPVEHH
Electrophorus	SEDETRLVKLNFSGYNKVVRPVNHF

conserved   ** ** *   *   ***

Fig. 1

Each subunit is transmembrane and the pentameric complex $\alpha_2\beta\gamma\delta$ constitutes a complete physiological receptor for postsynaptic depolarization containing both the binding sites for the neurotransmitter and the ion channel opened in response to AcCh binding (see Conti-Tronconi and Raftery 1982).

2. Non-equivalence of the Two α-Subunits

Each α-subunit has a high affinity binding site for cholinergic ligands but the two sites are not equivalent. Bromoacetylcholine can be used to label one or both α-subunits while MBTA labels only one (see Conti-Tronconi and Raftery 1982). The non-equivalence of these two sites can be explained by their different microenvironments since each α-chain must be flanked by different subunits. In addition, the two α-subunits could be chemically different, in spite of their identical primary structure. The α-subunits of the *Torpedo* AChR have been purified by preparative SDS gel electrophoresis and after proteolysis using V8 protease two prominent peptides of $M_r \sim 17,000$ and 19,000 were present in similar amounts (Conti-Tronconi et al. 1984a). It had previously been reported (Gullick et al. 1981) that only the 19K peptide can be labeled by MBTA under mild reducing conditions and that only the 17K peptide can be stained for carbohydrates. We have determined the amino terminal sequence of all the peptides obtained after V8 digestion and found that the 17K and 19K peptides had the same NH_2-terminal sequence starting at residue 47. Since even extensive proteolysis does not convert the 19K peptide to the 17K peptide. These results indicate that the two α-chains differ in their extent of glycosylation, the binding site on the less glycosylated α-subunit is likely to be more accessible to reducing and affinity labeling reagents, thus explaining the non-equivalence of high affinity ligand binding to the two subunits.

3. Is the Torpedo AChR a Good Model for Other Nicotinic AChRs?

Study of the AChR from other sources has been hampered by difficulties in obtaining suitable amounts of intact AChR, due to the much lower AChR content and to high levels of protease activity. Similarities in the pharmacology, morphology, antigenicity, and physical properties as well as the frequent presence upon $NaDoDSO_4$ gel electrophoresis of complex polypeptide patterns (see Conti-Tronconi and Raftery 1982), reminiscent of the subunit pattern of *Torpedo* AChR, suggests the likelihood of close structural and functional similarities between the AChRs from different sources.

Torpedo (a marine elasmobranch) and *Electrophorus* (a freshwater teleost) are highly diverged species whose evolution arose separately from the primordial vertebrate stock (~ 400 million years ago) and accordingly the presence of electric organs in these two species is due to convergent evolution. The purified AChR from *Electrophorus* electric organ contains four main polypeptides in the same M_r range of *Torpedo* AChR. For each of the four peptides, the amino terminal amino acid sequence was determined (Conti-Tronconi et al. 1982a; Fig. 1). The four subunits have distinct but homologous sequences and the degree of identity between pairs of subunits ranges between 47.5% and 37.5%. Numerous conservative substitutions tend to further increase the degree of similarity among subunits. Furthermore the sequences are homologous (up to 62.5% identity) to those of *Torpedo* AChR subunits of comparable M_r. Simultaneous quantitative sequencing of the peptides present in preparations of intact *Electrophorus* AChR was used to determine the subunit stoichiometry (Table 1). Molar ratios of 2:1:1:1 were obtained for the subunits of M_r 41,000 (α_1), 50,000 (β_1), 55,000 (γ_1) and 62,000 (δ_1), respectively.

Upon SDS gel electrophoresis of AChR from *Electrophorus* muscle four main polypeptides were observed whose molecular weights were similar but not identical to the molecular weights of the four peptides present in the electric organ AChR. Each of these peptides has been isolated and their amino terminal sequences have been determined. Again the AChRs from muscle were found to be composed of four homologous proteins of apparent molecular weight 40,500, 50,000, 56,000 and 63,000, respectively.

Table 1. AChR subunit stoichiometry of *Torpedo californica* electric organ

Subunit	Residues			Triton-solubilized AChR[a]		Membrane-bound AChR[a]	
				Preparation 1	Preparation 2	Preparation 3	Preparation 4
α	Ala-9	Asn-10	Asn-14	1.93 ± 0.13	1.92 ± 0.14	1.96 ± 0.04	2.05 ± 0.16
β	Ser-9	Val-10	Thr-14	1.02 ± 0.08	1.07 ± 0.09	1.03 ± 0.04	1.02 ± 0.01
γ	Glu-9	Lys-10	Asp-14	1.00 ± 0.10	1.02 ± 0.21	1.01 ± 0.03	1.00 ± 0.07
δ	Asn-9	Asp-10	Val-14	1.04 ± 0.07	1.00 ± 0.13	1.01 ± 0.08	0.93 ± 0.08

Average

α	1.97 ± 0.12
β	1.03 ± 0.06
γ	1.01 ± 0.10
δ	0.99 ± 0.09

Electrophorus electricus electric organ

Subunit	Residues		Preparation 1	Preparation 2	Average of 1 and 2
α_1	Val-8,	Gly-14	1.90 ± 0.19	1.96 ± 0.18	1.93 ± 0.10
β_1	Met-8,	Ala-14	1.02 ± 0.02	0.99 ± 0.01	1.01 ± 0.02
γ_1	Ala-8,	Tyr-14	1.10 ± 0.27	1.04 ± 0.12	1.08 ± 0.20
δ_1	Ile-8,	Glu-14	1.02 ± 0.07	1.00 ± 0.05	1.04 ± 0.06

Mammalian Muscle (fetal calf)

Subunit	Residue (cycle 8)	Ratio
α	Val-8	2.16
β	Leu-8	0.95
x	Gln-8	0.92
y	Ile-8	0.98

[a] Values are means ± SEM

No difference was found between the sequenced segments of corresponding subunits from muscle and from electric organ AChR.

To elucidate the structure of mammalian muscle AChR we purified the receptor from fetal calf muscle. Upon SDS gel electrophoresis the purified AChR resolved into five major polypeptides having molecular weights (M_r) of 42, 44, 49, 55 and 58K. The peptide of M_r 44K is actin because it contains 3-methyl-histidine and binds anti-actin antibodies and the peptide of M_r 42K is labeled by (^{3}H)bromoacetylcholine (Conti-Tronconi et al. 1982b). Three subunits (M_r 42K, 49K and 53K) yielded distinct but homologous sequences. Due to the lack of identifiable sequences associated with the 55K and 58K polypeptides (most likely due to blockage of their amino terminals during isolation) intact AChR preparations were analysed. Four homologous sequences were obtained (Fig. 1). Three were identical with those independently determined and the fourth sequence could be deduced by difference. The four sequences were present in a stoichiometry of 2:1:1:1 (Table 1) which demonstrates that like electric fish AChR mammalian muscle nicotinic receptor is a pentameric complex composed of two equivalent and three pseudoequivalent subunits.

Recently we have purified the AChR from denervated chick muscle. As for the AChRs from other receptor species a multi-subunit pattern was observed. The amino terminal sequence of the α-subunit (Fig. 1; Barnard et al. 1983) is again homologous to the α-subunits of the receptor from other species and we have further demonstrated that this receptor also is composed of four homologous subunits in the ratio $\alpha_2\beta\gamma\delta$.

4. Brain AChR

Some regions of the vertebrate brain contain a nicotinic AChR with pharmacological characteristics similar but not identical to those of muscle AChR. In addition, some brain areas and peripheral ganglia contain high affinity binding sites for α-bungarotoxin (α-BTX) and similar snake toxins, which are known to bind to peripheral AChR. However, the identity of the neuronal toxin-binding component with a nicotinic AChR has been disputed since in some areas of the brain α-BuTx does not always block receptor function (see Barnard et al. 1983). Using procedures designed to minimize AChR proteolysis we have isolated the AChR from chick optic lobe and the rest of the brain by affinity chromatography. The peptide composition of the optic lobe AChR displays somehow characteristics similar to those of the peripheral AChRs. All the peptides contained in purified optic lobe AChR were isolated and submitted to amino terminal amino acid sequencing. Amino terminal sequence analysis of the higher M_r subunits from optic lobe AChR did not yield any signal above the high background consistently present, indicating that these subunits had blocked NH_2 termini. However, the lowest M_r component gave a readily identifiable single sequence, reported in Fig. 1. Comparison of this sequence with the known amino terminal sequences of *Torpedo*, *Electrophorus* and calf peripheral AChR subunits, the α-subunit of chick and the other subunits of chick muscle AChR (unpublished observations) revealed that the optic lobe sequence is, although different, highly homologous to the subunits of the other AChRs, the highest degree of homology being with the α-subunits and among these with the α-subunit of *Torpedo* (see Fig. 1). This would indicate that the divergence of peripheral and central nicotinic receptors happened very early during vertebrate evolution.

These results establish that the CNS α-bungarotoxin binding protein is indeed a nicotinic receptor similar to those found in muscle and electric organ. Brain and muscle AChR from the same species, although homologous, must be encoded by different genes and must have originated from the same ancestral gene. Since the similarity between α-subunits of central and peripheral receptors from the same animal is much less than between α-subunits of peripheral AChRs from different animals it may be concluded that the central and peripheral nicotinic receptors diverged very early during vertebrate evolution. These divergencies from common ancestral structure explain well the pharmacological characteristics of these receptors which only partially overlap.

References

Barnard EA, Beeson D, Bilbe G, Brown DA, Constanti A, Conti-Tronconi BM, Dolly JO, Dunn SMJ, Mehraban F, Richards GM, Smart TG (1983) Cold Spring Harbor Symp Quant Biol 48: 109–124

Conti-Tronconi BM, Raftery MA (1982) Annu Rev Biochem 51:491

Conti-Tronconi BM, Hunkapiller MW, Lindstrom JM, Raftery MA (1982a) Proc Natl Acad Sci USA 79:6489

Conti-Tronconi BM, Gotti C, Hunkapiller MW, Raftery MA (1982b) Science 218:1227

Conti-Tronconi BM, Hunkapiller MW, Raftery MA (1984a) Proc Natl Acad Sci USA 81:2631

Conti-Tronconi BM, Hunkapiller MW, Lindstrom JM, Raftery MA (1984b) J Recept Res 4:801–816

Conti-Tronconi BM, Dunn SMJ, Barnard EA, Dolly JO, Lai FA, Ray N, Raftery MA (1985) Proc Natl Acad Sci USA (in press)

Gullick W, Tzartos S, Lindstrom J (1981) Biochemistry 20:2173

Martinez-Carrion M, Sator V, Raftery MA (1975) Biochem Biophys Res Commun 65:129

Noda M, Takahashi H, Tanabe T, Toyosato M, Kikyotani S, Furotani Y, Hirose T, Takashima H, Mayama S, Miyata T, Numa S (1983) Nature 30:528

Raftery MA, Hunkapiller MW, Strader CD, Hood LE (1980) Science 208:1454

Structure and Function of the Nicotinic Acetylcholine Receptor and of the Voltage-dependent Na$^+$-Channel

M.A. RAFTERY, B.M. CONTI-TRONCONI, and S.M.J. DUNN[1]

1. Introduction

Nicotinic acetylcholine receptors (AChRs) from electric organs and muscle of different species have been shown to be highly conserved proteins composed of four homologous subunits occurring in the stoichiometry $\alpha_2\beta\gamma\delta$ and forming a pseudosymmetric penta-meric complex (see Raftery et al. 1983). The availability of large quantities of AChR from *Torpedo* electric organ has greatly facilitated detailed studies of its structure and function. It has been demonstrated that the $\alpha_2\beta\gamma\delta$ complex constitutes the complete physiological receptor for postsynaptic depolarization by ACh and contains both the binding sites for cholinergic ligands and the cation gating unit (Moore and Raftery 1980; Wu et al. 1981). Each subunit spans the postsynaptic membrane and each has been shown to be exposed to the lipid bilayer suggesting that all subunits may interact with the surrounding membrane in a related fashion (see Raftery et al. 1983).

2. Cation Gating Function of AChR

Correlation of the subunit structure of the AChR with its physiological function necessitates the development of quantitative methods to evaluate the efficiency of receptor mediated cation transport in vitro. A rapid kinetic method was developed for this purpose to allow spectroscopic detection of monovalent cation transport (Moore and Raftery 1980). A water soluble fluorophore (8-aminonaphthalene 1,3,6 tri-sulfonate, ANTS) is trapped within AChR enriched vesicles and the quench of its fluorescence caused by agonist mediated inward transport of thallium (I) ion is moni-tored in stopped-flow experiments, allowing detection of transport on a millisecond time scale. The rate of fluorescence decay depends on the number of activated AChRs and this can be used to determine the level of ion transport mediated by a single AChR molecule. Using this approach Moore and Raftery (1980) showed that the maximum rate at high Carb concentrations corresponds to transport of 7×10^6 ions

---

1   The Braun Laboratories of the Division of Chemistry, California Institute of Technology, Pasadena, CA 91125, USA

Molecular Aspects of Neurobiology
(ed. by Rita Levi Montalcini et al.)
© Springer-Verlag Berlin Heidelberg 1986

per second per receptor in *Torpedo* Ringers which is very close to that estimated for AChR at the neuromuscular junction in vivo, demonstrating that the receptor in isolated vesicles is fully functional. Reconstitution studies using detergent solubilized AChR preparations where the AChR polypeptides were the only protein components reassociated with phospholipid vesicles (Wu et al. 1981) have demonstrated that the specific cation transport rate per AChR molecule was within a factor of two of those reported earlier for native membrane preparations (Moore and Raftery 1980). This confirm that only the four receptor polypeptides ($\alpha, \beta, \gamma, \delta$) are necessary to form the active complex. In these ion flux assays the midpoint of the dose response for Carb-mediated flux occurs at ~ 1 mM and for ACh at $\sim 100\,\mu$M. Such high concentrations of agonist necessary for activation of ion transport are in agreement with electrophysiological studies but at variance with many direct studies of ligand binding to AChR in either the resting or desensitized state. Another aspect of the flux response is that for ACh it is a cooperative phenomenon with a Hill coefficient of 1.7 (Raftery et al. 1983).

3. Ligand Binding to AChR

The AChR complex contains binding sites for several types of ligands including agonists, cholinergic antagonists, polypeptide neurotoxins, small molecule neurotoxins and local anesthetics (Conti-Tronconi and Raftery 1982). Some but not all of these ligands compete for the same binding sites and therefore multiple receptor-ligand associations are possible. This leads to more complex models of such interactions than generally considered.

Measurements of the equilibrium binding of agonists to the AChR have shown that under these conditions in which the receptor is desensitized and the ion channel is closed, the affinity for agonists is high (Kd ~ 10 nM for ACh). Since channel opening occurs within a few milliseconds of neurotransmitter release functionally important conformational changes must occur on rapid time scales. A variety of stopped-flow fluorescence techniques have therefore been used to investigate the interaction of agonists with AChR under pre-equilibrium conditions (see Conti-Tronconi and Raftery 1982). In all early reports of such rapid kinetic studies there are two major problems in correlating any observed receptor conformation change with the open channel state: (1) apparent dissociation constants for agonist binding to the resting state of the AChR are lower than those obtained from the concentration dependence of the permeability response; and (2) no observed conformational change is fast enough to be identified with channel opening which must occur on a millisecond time scale. It is therefore likely that these slow processes are related to desensitization or other inactivation mechanisms which in electrophysiological experiments have been shown to occur on similar time scales.

A high affinity binding site for agonists has been assigned to each α-subunit since following reduction of a reactive disulphide bond near the site it can be labeled by affinity alkylating agents such as bromoacetylcholine (see Conti-Tronconi and Raftery 1982). Equilibrium binding constants calculated from the kinetic parameters measured in the stopped-flow studies suggest that in these experiments the binding of agonists to these α-subunit sites was measured and it is notable that observed conformational changes were all too slow to be primary events in channel activation.

It has generally been assumed that the well-characterized sites on the α-subunits are the only binding sites for agonists and that their occupancy leads in a sequential manner to both functional responses of channel opening and desensitization. Recently, however, we have demonstrated the existence of a low affinity site(s) for agonists which is present under equilibrium conditions and which is distinct from the high affinity sites which can be labeled by bromoacetylcholine (Conti-Tronconi et al. 1982; Dunn and Raftery 1982a,b; Dunn et al. 1983). The characteristics of agonist binding to the low affinity site(s) suggest their involvement in channel activation.

The membrane-bound AChR was covalently labeled by the fluorescence probe, IANBD without any impairment of function and it was shown that the fluorescence of this probe was enhanced in a saturable manner by the binding of agonists (Dunn and Raftery 1982a,b) with the same dose dependency as the flux response giving kds for Carb and ACh binding of $\sim$ 1 mM and $\sim$ 100 μM, respectively. Kinetic experiments have shown that the fluorescence change is a monophasic process occurring on a rapid time scale; the rate had a hyperbolic dependence on agonist concentration and the transition must therefore be a conformational change of the receptor-ligand complex, reaching a maximum rate of $\sim$ 400 s^{-1} for Carb and $\sim$ 600 s^{-1} for ACh.

The low affinity site(s) is distinct from the high affinity sites on the α-subunits since even when these latter sites were maximally labeled by BrACh, the fluorescence enhancement and therefore agonist binding to the low affinity site was unaltered (Conti-Tronconi et al. 1982; Dunn et al. 1983). In the presence of covalently bound BrACh no ion flux was observed. The conformational change occurring on agonist binding to the low affinity site is therefore independent of other transitions which inhibit channel opening.

Several lines of evidence implicate the low affinity site in channel opening and suggest that activation and desensitization are parallel pathways which are mediated by agonist binding to different sites: (1) the fluorescence enhancement is specific for agonists, is abolished by prior incubation with α-bungarotoxin and it reflects a conformational transition of the receptor-agonist complex; (2) kd values for agonist binding correspond to those for activation (Table 1); (3) the conformational change is rapid, reaching $\sim$ 400 s^{-1} for Carb and $\sim$ 600 s^{-1} for ACh; (4) Q_{10} is $\sim$ 2.5, in agreement with electrophysiological measurements for channel opening; and (5) the binding is unaffected by desensitization, covalently bound bromoacetylcholine or prior incubation with physiologically active concentrations of curare, HTX or local anesthetics.

4. Direct Binding Measurements to a Low Affinity Site

Recently we have been able to directly measure low affinity binding of a cholinergic agonist (^{3}H)suberyldicholine to the AChR. At low ligand concentration two high affinity sites for this ligand can be observed with kd $\sim$ 10 nM. However, at higher ligand concentration (in the μM range) a binding site with kd $\sim$ 0.6 μM can be observed

Table 1. Effect of agonists on fluorescence of NBD-labeled AChR and comparison with kd values from thallium flux data

Agonist	kd (Fluorescence), mM	kd (Thallium flux), mM[a]
SdCh[b]	0.001 ± 0.0005	0.001 ± 0.0007
ACh	0.09 ± 0.02	0.057
Carb	0.96 ± 0.17	1.0
Nicotine	0.60 ± 0.21	0.13
PTA	0.47 ± 0.09	0.11
Choline	∿ 35	–

[a] Data fitted to model where two ligand binding sites must be occupied for channel to open

$$k_{app} = \frac{k_{max} \ [L]^2}{(kd + [L])^2}$$

[b] SdCh, suberoyldicholine; ACh, acetylcholine; Carb, carbamoylcholine; PTA, phenyltrimethyl-ammonium ion

under equilibrium conditions. This agrees nicely with the dose-response curve for suberyldicholine which gives an apparent kd of 1 μM. These studies corroborate our observations with NBD-labeled AChR and provide strong support for our ideas of independent sites controlling activation and desensitization. The direct binding studies with (^{3}H)suberyldicholine (kd ∿ 1 μM) were not previously possible using (^{3}H) ACh or (^{3}H) carb since their kd values for binding to the low affinity site(s) are 75 μM and 1 μM, respectively, whereas the effective concentration of sites obtained in our preparations is maximally 10 μM.

Torpedo AChR therefore appears to have two classes of agonist binding sites – those of high affinity on the α-subunits which may be labeled by bromoacetylcholine and those of low affinity which are revealed by NBD fluorescence changes. The conformational change occurring on agonist binding to the low affinity site is unaffected by desensitization or by covalent labeling by bromoacetylcholine and the two pathways must therefore be independent. Such a model is illustrated pictorially in Fig. 1. In the resting state the "activation gate" is closed but in the presence of high concentrations of agonists the low affinity sites are occupied and the AChR undergoes a rapid conformational transition to an open channel state. Over longer time scales slow conformational transitions in another part of the molecule mediated by agonist binding to other sites, probably those of high equilibrium affinity on the α-subunits, cause the channel to close. Alternatively, at lower concentrations of agonist, occupancy of these latter sites causes slow conformational changes which close an "inactivation gate." Under these circumstances the same conformational change may be induced by agonist binding to the low affinity sites but this transition cannot now lead to opening of the ion channel.

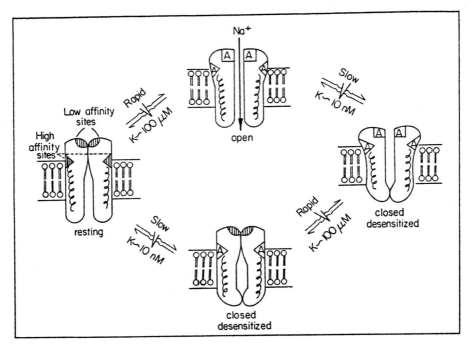

Fig. 1

5. Voltage-Dependent Sodium Channel

The sodium channel is also an integral membrane protein containing an ion channel, but its ion gating properties are modulated by changes in the transmembrane voltage. This protein from *Electrophorus electricus* is formed by a single, large peptide of $M_r \sim 250{,}000$ and its complete primary structure has recently been elucidated by cloning and sequence analysis of cDNA (Noda et al. 1984). The sodium channel is composed of 1820 amino acid residues and has four internal repeats that exhibit sequence homology, suggesting that these four units have evolved from a single common ancestor by gene duplications. Each homology unit contains a unique positively charged segment as well as four clusters of negatively charged residues between the second and third homology units which have been assigned to the cytoplasmic side of the membrane (Noda et al. 1984). It is attractive to hypothesize that each of the four positively charged segments, possibly in conjunction with each of the four negatively charged segments, acts as voltage sensor, thus being involved in an activation gate.

References

Conti-Tronconi BM, Raftery MA (1982) Annu Rev Biochem 51:491

Conti-Tronconi BM, Dunn SMJ, Raftery MA (1982) Biochem Biophys Res Commun 107:123

Dunn SMJ, Raftery MA (1982a) Proc Natl Acad Sci USA 79:6757

Dunn SMJ, Raftery MA (1982b) Biochemistry 21:6264

Dunn SMJ, Conti-Tronconi BM, Raftery MA (1983) Biochemistry 22:2512

Moore HPH, Raftery MA (1980) Proc Natl Acad Sci USA 77:4509

Noda M, Shimizu S, Tanabe T, Takai T, Kayano T, Ideda T, Takahashi H, Nakayama H, Kanaoka Y, Minamino N, Kangawa K, Matsuo H, Raftery MA, Hiorse T, Knayama S, Hayashida H, Miyata T, Numa S (1984) Nature 312:121

Raftery MA, Dunn SMJ, Conti-Tronconi BM, Middlemas DS, Crawford RD (1983) Cold Spring Harbor Symp Quant Biol 48:181

Wu WCS, Moore HPH, Raftery MA (1981) Proc Natl Acad Sci USA 78:775

Molecular Cloning of Receptors for Acetylcholine

J. BOULTER, K. EVANS, S. EVANS, P. GARDNER, D. GOLDMAN,
S. HEINEMANN, W. LUYTEN, G. MARTIN, P. MASON, J. PATRICK,
and D. TRECO[1]

1. Introduction

The nicotinic acetylcholine receptor at the vertebrate neuromuscular junction has provided an excellent model both for studies of ligand-gated ion channels and for studies of neural regulation of the synthesis and properties of constituents of the neuromuscular junction. Research in many laboratories studying the biochemical and biophysical properties of the receptor has led to our current view of the receptor molecule (for review see Cold Spring Harbor Symposium on Quantitative Biology, Vol. XLVIII). The results of this research have also provided the basis for another more recent assault on the structure and regulation of the acetylcholine receptor. In this work the emphasis has been on the isolation of recombinant DNA molecules coding for the polypeptides that comprise the receptor oligomer. The nucleotide sequences of these DNA molecules provided the amino acid sequence of each of the four receptor subunits (Noda et al. 1983) and analysis of these sequences has provided support for various models for the disposition of receptor sequences across the membrane (Claudio et al. 1983) and for the location (Noda et al. 1983) of the acetylcholine binding site.

In addition to providing new insights and testable hypotheses about receptor structure these receptor coding sequences have permitted new access to neural regulation of the properties and synthesis of acetylcholine receptor. Innervated muscle produces a receptor molecule that is distinguishable biochemically and functionally from that made by a muscle following denervation. In addition, acetylcholine receptor is much more abundant on denervated muscle than on innervated muscle due to a greater rate of synthesis (Merlie et al. 1977). It is now clear that the increased rate of synthesis of the α-subunit is due at least in part to an increase in the abundance of α-subunit coding mRNA species (Merlie et al. 1983a,b; Goldman et al. 1985). Furthermore, the mRNA made following denervation is indistinguishable by S1 analysis throughout its protein-coding sequence from the mRNA made by innervated muscle (Goldman et al. 1985). This suggests that the differences in properties between the receptors in innervated and denervated muscle are due either to a post-translational modification or to differences attributable to the other receptor subunits. Furthermore, a non-fusing muscle cell line

---

[1] The Salk Institute, P.O. Box 85800, San Diego, CA 92138, USA

Molecular Aspects of Neurobiology
(ed. by Rita Levi Montalcini et al.)
© Springer-Verlag Berlin Heidelberg 1986

BC_3H-1 produces acetylcholine receptor only after cessation of cell division (Patrick et al. 1977). Yet this cell line makes mRNA coding for the α-subunit of the receptor while in the logarithmic phase of growth (Merlie et al. 1983) suggesting that post-transcriptional events regulate the appearance of receptor on the cell surface. The availability of cDNA clones coding for the mouse (BC_3H-1) nicotinic acetylcholine receptor may provide the means of understanding the various mechanisms of regulating the appearance of functional acetylcholine receptor molecules.

There are nicotinic acetylcholine receptors on nerve cells that differ from those found on either innervated or denervated muscle. The structure and biochemical properties of these receptors are less well understood largely because the molecules have not been as readily accessible. The toxins that provided such powerful tools for the study of the muscle type nicotinic receptor are of uncertain value for study of the neural type nicotinic receptor (Patrick et al. 1977). The degree to which neural regulation of muscle nicotinic receptors can be extrapolated to neural regulation of receptors at nerve-nerve synapses is not known. If sufficient homology exists between the two types of nicotinic receptors it may be possible to use DNA sequences coding for the muscle nicotinic receptor to isolate clones coding for the nerve type nicotinic receptor. This access, through the genome, to neural receptor molecules might bypass the difficult steps of protein purification and analysis.

2. Isolation of Clones Coding for Mouse Muscle (BC_3H-1) Acetylcholine Receptor

The non-fusing mouse muscle cell line is a rich source of the muscle nicotinic acetylcholine receptor. The receptor is abundant on the cell surface and is rapidly metabolized ($t_{1/2} \sim 8$ h) suggesting that the cells have a high capacity for receptor synthesis and might be a good source of mRNA coding for receptor subunits (Patrick et al. 1977). We purified mRNA from this cell line and constructed two cDNA libraries, one in pBR322 and one in λ gt$_{10}$, from which we have obtained cDNA clones coding for the entire mature α (Boulter et al. 1985), β and γ-subunits of mouse muscle acetylcholine receptor. A cDNA clone coding for the entire δ-subunit has been isolated from a cDNA library prepared from BC_3H-1 mRNA (La Polla et al. 1985) and cDNA clone coding for the carboxy terminal sequences of the BC_3H-1 receptor was isolated by Merlie (1983).

Clone pMARα15 was isolated from a cDNA library prepared in pBR322 (Boulter et al. 1985). A library of 50,000 elements was screened with a genomic fragment containing sequences coding for a portion of the chick muscle receptor α-subunit (Ballivet et al. 1983). Two positive clones were obtained one of which, pMARα15, contained an insert of about 1700 base pairs. The insert in pMARα15 was sequenced and found to contain the entire coding region of the mature protein. It also codes for an additional 8 amino acids 5' to the amino terminus. Since these amino acids are all uncharged, they are probably part of an incomplete signal peptide. The clone does not contain an ATG codon 5' to the amino terminus of the mature protein. The 3' untranslated sequences contain three possible polyadenylation sites, one at position 1552 and two overlapping sequences around position 1675. As discussed below, both these polyadenylation sites are used. The protein encoded by pMARα15 contains 437 amino acids and is 78% homologous with *Torpedo,* 94% homologous with the muscle acetylcholine receptor α-subunit of human and calf.

Clones coding for the mouse muscle acetylcholine receptor were also isolated from a cDNA library prepared in λ gt$_{10}$. This library had a base of 10^6 elements and was screened after amplification with a sequence coding for a portion of the *Torpedo* β-subunit which we obtained from K. Mixter and N. Davidson. From this initial screening, we obtained about 10^2 hybridizing plaques out of 10^6 plaques that we examined. Phage from these plaques were purified and the size of the insert DNA was determined. We chose one clone with an insert of about 2000 bp for sequence analysis and discovered that the sequences coded for proteins that were more similar to the γ-subunit than to the β-subunit. In fact, we later found that the majority of the clones identified by the *Torpedo* β-subunit probe coded for mouse γ sequences. We subsequently devised an assay based on known restriction sites in the mouse γ and δ-subunits and re-examined the clones we identified with the *Torpedo* β-subunit probe. This second screening produced clones that were neither γ nor δ and which contained sequences having extensive homology with the *Torpedo* and calf muscle β-subunits.

A clone, pMARγ144, has been sequenced and found to code for the entire mature γ-subunit of mouse muscle (BC$_3$H-1) acetylcholine receptor. The clone contains 1786 base pairs and has an open reading frame of 1491 base pairs which codes for a protein of 497 amino acids with a calculated molecular weight of 56,400 daltons. The clone also contains sequences at the 5′ end that code for a portion of the signal peptide. None of our γ coding cDNA clones isolated to date have sequences coding for a complete signal peptide. It is not the case, however, that the most 5′ sequences in the clone code for the partial signal peptide. In general, the most 5′ sequences do not appear to code for a receptor precursor and are of unknown origin. This is also the case for several of our clones coding for the mouse muscle α and γ-subunits. In each case, the identifiable receptor coding sequence stops at a string of leucine residues present in the leader sequence of many mammalian receptor subunits, perhaps because the high GC content of this region interferes with further accurate synthesis by the reverse transcriptase.

Clones containing sequences coding for the α or γ-subunit contain two polyadenylation signals and it is likely that both these signals are used during processing of the transcript in muscle. In the case of the α-subunit we find two mRNA species that differ in length by about 150 bases; Sl nuclease mapping demonstrates that the two species differ at the 3′ end (Goldman et al. 1985). The two polyadenylation sites in pMARα15 are separated by about 150 bases. We have isolated two classes of γ coding cDNA clones that differ by 200 bases at their 3′ ends. The class with the additional 3′ sequences has a polyadenylation site about 200 bases from the 3′ end. Furthermore, the clone with the shorter 3′ untranslated sequence does have an oligo (A) tract showing that both of the polyadenylation signals are used. Like the α-coding clone, the γ coding clone identifies two mRNA species that differ in size by an amount equal to the difference in 3′ untranslated sequences. It does not appear that either of the two sites is used preferentially in denervated or innervated muscle.

3. Analysis of Receptor Coding mRNA in Innervated and Denervated Muscle

Denervation of skeletal muscle results in an increase in the abundance of receptor coding mRNA (Merlie et al. 1983a,b; Goldman et al. 1985). Denervation of mouse leg muscle produces about a 50-fold increase in the abundance of the α-subunit coding mRNA and a similar increase in mRNA species coding for the β, γ and δ-subunits. However, denervation of rat diaphragm produces only a 7-fold increase in the abundance of mRNA coding for the α-subunit. It is not clear why the increase in abundance of α-subunit coding mRNA of rat diaphragm is less than that of mouse leg muscle.

The α-subunit mRNA species found before and after denervation of mouse leg muscle are indistinguishable by S1 nuclease mapping (Goldman et al. 1985). pMARα15 was subcloned in phage M13 and the corresponding single strand DNAs prepared. The mRNA from both innervated and denervated muscle protected the entirety of this sequence from digestion with nuclease S1. We have not, however, ruled out the possibility that there are differences in the 5' portion of the signal peptide or in the 5' untranslated sequences. However, our present results fail to provide any evidence for differences between the α-subunit coding mRNA species made before or after denervation and suggest that a single gene codes for the α-subunit made in both circumstances. In this case, the several differences seen between junctional and extrajunctional acetylcholine receptor might be due either to differences in the amino acid sequence of one of the other subunits or to post-translational modification of any of the four subunits.

4. Identification in Nerve Cells of Sequences Homologous to Muscle Acetylcholine Receptor

The nicotinic acetylcholine receptor on ganglionic neurons shares properties with, but is distinguishable from, the nicotinic acetylcholine receptor on muscle. For example, the snake toxin, α-bungarotoxin, binds to and blocks function of the receptor on muscle but has no effect on the activation of the receptor on PC12 cells (Patrick and Stallcup 1977). There is, however, a toxin-binding component on nerve cells which is distinguishable from the acetylcholine receptor by its reaction with antibodies (Patrick and Stallcup 1977), its localization (Jacob and Berg 1983) and its regulation (Mitsuka and Hatanake 1983; Smith et al. 1983). Since purification of either the toxin-binding component or the nerve type nicotinic receptor from nerve cells is difficult, we have tried to identify DNA sequences coding for either of these components by hybridization with DNA sequences coding for the muscle nicotinic acetylcholine receptor.

A radioactive probe prepared from clone pMARα15 hybridizes to mRNA species present in poly (A)$^+$ RNA made from rat brain or the PC12 pheochromocytoma cell line. The hybrids are not stable during high stringency washing (0.1 × SSPE, 65°C) indicating that the RNA species identified by pMARα15 are not identical to pMARα15. We prepared cDNA from mRNA isolated from the PC12 cell line, inserted this cDNA into the Eco RI site of λgt$_{10}$, and made a library of 5 × 10^6 elements. The library was screened at low stringency with a probe made from pMARα15 and three hybridiz-ing phage were purified from 10^6 examined. One of these clones, pPCα48, has sequence homology with pMARα15 and might therefore code for either the ganglionic nicotinic acetylcholine receptor or the toxin-binding component found on nerve cells. The same library was screened with a radioactive probe prepared from the clones coding for the β and γ-subunits of mouse muscle nicotinic receptor. In each case, hybridizing clones were identified and purified.

Since the sequences in clone pPCα48 were derived from rat and were identified by mouse sequences, the lack of high stringency hybridization might be a consequence only of species differences. In this case pPCα48, although isolated from the PC12 cell line, might code for the rat muscle nicotinic receptor. We tested this possibility by forming heteroduplexes between a single strand of pPCα48 and mRNA isolated from PC12 or rat denervated muscle. The PC12 RNA but not the rat diaphragm RNA protected pPCα48 from digestion with nuclease Sl. This result suggests that pPCα48 does not code for the rat muscle nicotinic receptor.

5. Summary

Various snake neurotoxins and the electric organs of electric fishes and eels have greatly facilitated biochemical analysis of the muscle type nicotinic acetylcholine receptor. This early biochemical work provided information and reagents that were essential for the isolation of recombinant cDNA molecules with sequences coding for the subunits of *Torpedo* acetylcholine receptor. These clones have provided both the primary structure of the acetylcholine receptor and access to the acetylcholine recep-tor synthesized by mammalian muscle. Clones coding for mouse muscle acetylcholine receptor subunits isolated by hybridization with clones coding for *Torpedo* receptor subunits, yielded the primary structure of the mammalian receptor subunits. These clones in turn have identified related sequences in the central and peripheral nervous system that may provide the primary structure for a variety of acetylcholine receptors or related proteins. This approach to the components of the nervous system is thus valuable both because of its capacity to reveal related proteins and because it may circumvent the need to purify these proteins.

References

Ballivet M, Nef P, Stalder R, Fulpius B (1983) Cold Spring Harbor Symp Quant Biol 48:83–87
Boulter J, Luyten W, Evans K, Mason P, Ballivet M, Goldman D, Martin G, Heinemann S, Patrick J (1985) J Neurosci 5:2545–2552
Claudio T, Ballivet M, Patrick J, Heinemann S (1983) Proc Natl Acad Sci 80:1111–1115
Goldman D, Boulter J, Heinemann S, Patrick J (1985) J Neurosci 5:2553–2558
Jacob MH, Berg DK (1983) J Neurosci 3:260–271
La Polla RJ, Mixter-Mayne K, Davidson N (1984) Proc Natl Acad Sci USA 81:7970–7974

Merlie JP, Sebbane R, Gardner S, Lindstrom J (1983a) Proc Natl Acad Sci 80:3845

Merlie JP, Sebbane R, Gardner S, Olson E, Lindstrom J (1983b) Cold Spring Harbor Symp Quant Biol XLVII 135

Mitsuka M, Hatanake H (1983) J Neurosci 3:1785

Noda M, Takahashi H, Tanabe T, Toxosato M, Kikyotani S, Furutani Y, Hirose T, Takashima H, Inyama S, Miyata T, Numa W (1983) Nature (Lond) 302:528–532

Patrick J, Stallcup W (1977) Proc Natl Acad Sci 74:4689

Patrick J, McMillan J, Wolfson M, O'Brien JC (1977) J Biol Chem 252:2143

Smith MA, Margiotta JF, Berg DK (1983) J Neurosci 3:2395–2407

The Molecular Biology of Acetylcholine Receptors from the Vertebrate Peripheral and Central Nervous Systems

J.F. JACKSON[1], D.M.W. BEESON[1,2], V.B. COCKCROFT[1], M.G. DARLISON[1], B.M. CONTI-TRONCONI[3], L.D. BELL[2], and E.A. BARNARD[1]

1. Introduction

Nicotinic acetylcholine receptors (AChR) mediate chemical communication at synapses in many parts of the vertebrate nervous system, including neuromuscular junctions, autonomic ganglia, and certain sites in the brain. This occurs through the interaction of neuronally-released acetylcholine (ACh) with recognition sites on the AChR in the postsynaptic membrane. ACh binding activates a gated cation channel and results in a transient change in the permeability of the membrane, which can be measured as a depolarisation of the transmembrane electrical potential. This has been directly demonstrated for the best characterised AChR, that from the electroplax of *Torpedo* sp. or *Electrophorus* sp. The *Torpedo* electric organ is a rich source of AChR protein and mRNA, and studies on this model system have contributed crucially to our understanding of AChR structure and function. An extensive review literature is available (Karlin 1980; Conti-Tronconi and Raftery 1982; Kistler et al. 1982; Dolly and Barnard 1984; Popot and Changeux 1984).

2. The Vertebrate Muscle AChR: A Homologous Protein

Though present at a concentration three orders of magnitude lower than that in the *Torpedo* electric organ, the vertebrate muscle AChR is very similar in structure and function. AChR purified from denervated chicken pectoral muscle (where the AChR concentration is 20–40-fold higher than in innervated muscle), when complexed with $[^{125}I]\alpha$-BuTX, cosediments with the 9S complex from *Torpedo*. SDS gel electrophoresis of this AChR shows the overall similarity to *Torpedo* AChR: a 43K alpha subunit which binds toxin and can be affinity labeled with bromoacetylcholine (Br-ACh); a 50K beta subunit, a 55K gamma subunit and a 57K delta subunit are

1 Department of Biochemistry, Imperial College of Science and Technology, London SW7 2AZ, U.K.
2 Searle Research and Development, PO Box 53, Lane End Road, High Wycombe, Buckinghamshire, HP12 4HL, U.K.
3 Division of Chemistry, California Institute of Technology, Pasadena, CA 91125, USA

Molecular Aspects of Neurobiology
(ed. by Rita Levi Montalcini et al.)
© Springer-Verlag Berlin Heidelberg 1986

present in the usual stoichiometry. Amino-terminal microsequence analysis demonstrates that each subunit is strongly homologous to the *Torpedo* counterpart (Beeson et al. 1985), and three of the four sequences have been confirmed by cloning (Nef et al. 1984; Beeson et al. 1985).

3. Chicken AChR Gene Cloning

The strong sequence conservation between vertebrate and fish AChR subunits permits isolation of vertebrate AChR genes from cDNA or genomic DNA libraries by cross-hybridization (Ballivet et al. 1983; Noda et al. 1983). In our hands, this strategy, in conjunction with rescreening using oligonucleotides derived from the amino terminus of the chicken α-subunit, yielded full-length cDNA clones from an embryonic pectoral muscle cDNA library (Beeson et al. 1986).

The 1812 nucleotide long sequence obtained contains a single long open reading frame which was used to deduce the complete amino acid sequence of the alpha subunit (Beeson et al. 1986). After a segment corresponding to the signal sequence, the deduced amino acid sequence was found to match the chemically determined N-terminal amino acid sequence. Only one difference (glu in the gene at position 14 instead of the asp predicted) is found between these two in the first 29 residues. The mature subunit has 437 residues, as do all three other fully sequenced alpha AChR genes (Noda et al. 1983) and a deduced molecular weight of 50,095 daltons. Using the same strategy, we have also isolated, but not completely sequenced, full-length cDNA clones corresponding to the other three subunits of this muscle AChR.

4. Receptor Biology

These DNA probes are being used in two studies which are currently in progress in our laboratories: (1) regulation of receptor biosynthesis during embryonic development and following denervation and (2) isolation of central nervous system AChR genes. Northern blots show that mature α-subunit mRNA from embryonic, denervated or normal muscle migrates as a single species of 3.1 kb. Upon longer exposure of the autoradiogram additional bands of 4.2 and 5.9 kb can be seen in all three lanes (unpublished observations). These larger species probably represent incompletely processed primary transcripts (nuclear RNA molecules containing unexcised intervening sequences) and have been noted by others (Takai et al. 1984). In any case, integration of densitometric scans of the autoradiogram reveal the three size classes are present in identical proportions in each of the three samples.

The extrajunctional AChR that appears upon denervation is known to be newly synthesised and not recruited from either a reserve pool of inactive receptor or by redistribution of synaptic receptor. Regulation of this new net synthesis could occur at one or more of many points. Insertion of AChR in the muscle plasma membrane is the last step in a long synthetic pathway which includes transcription of the four structural genes, processing and polyadenylation of nuclear RNA, transport of mRNA to the cytoplasm, translation of mRNA, co-translational modification within the rough endoplasmic reticulum, posttranslational modification within the Golgi apparatus and assembly of AChR subunits. Either by densitometric scans of Northern blots or "dot-blots", we find that denervation of chicken pectoral muscle results in an 20-fold increase in the steady-state level of α-subunit mRNA, as compared to normal pectoral muscle (unpublished observations). Messenger RNA yield per gram of tissue and mRNA purity, as assayed by hybridization to tritiated poly(U), is similar in all cases. Merlie et al. (1984), using Northern blot analysis, have reported a 100-fold increase in the steady-state level of mouse α-subunit mRNA following denervation of the hind limb. The reason for this discrepancy is not clear, but could simply reflect differences in the physiology of the muscles or organisms used. Since the increase in α-subunit mRNA observed upon denervation parallels that of the receptor protein as assayed by toxin binding, this accumulation is due either to mRNA stabilization, increased RNA transcription or both. Run-off assays using isolated nuclei can distinguish between these possibilities (Greenberg and Ziff 1984).

The absolute level of α-subunit sequences in denervated muscle mRNA, 0.017%, was derived by coelectrophoresis of denervated muscle mRNA with precisely measured amounts of pure rabbit globin mRNA (which migrates at 0.7 kb) followed by hybridization of the Northern blot with a 1:1 mixture of globin and AChR probes of identical specific activity. The abundance of AChR mRNA in innervated muscle can thus be calculated: AChR α-subunit mRNA, like the receptor protein, is present in innervated muscle at a concentration 3 logs lower than in *Torpedo* electroplax, 0.0009% versus 0.5% (unpublished observations).

5. AChR in the Central Nervous System?

Some regions of the vertebrate brain contain an AChR with pharmacological characteristics similar but not identical to those of muscle AChR (Morley and Kemp 1981; Oswald and Freeman 1981). Additionally, some brain areas and peripheral ganglia contain high affinity binding sites for α-BuTX. However, it is by no means generally accepted that the toxin binding components represent functional AChR. In amphibian and avian optic lobe (Oswald and Freeman 1981), human medulloblastoma cells (Syapin et al. 1982) and some sympathetic ganglion sites (Marshall 1981; Jacob and Berg 1983) there is evidence for this identity, even though α-BuTX binding does not always block receptor function. We (Norman et al. 1982) and others (Betz and Pfeiffer 1984) have isolated the α-BuTX does block AChR function (Oswald and Freeman 1981). We have conducted a series of experiments which indicate that the chicken optic lobe α-BuTX binding protein is an AChR structurally homologous to, but *significantly different* from peripheral AChR.

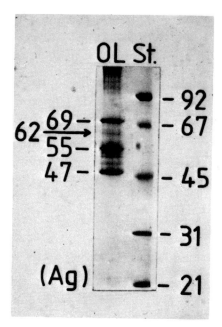

Fig. 1. Subunit composition of optic lobe AChR. Optic lobe AChR (*OL*) was electrophoresed on a SDS gel together with molecular weight markers (*St*). Proteins were visualized by silver staining. (From Conti-Tronconi et al. 1985)

6. The Optic Lobe AChR

Toxin-binding experiments detect α-BuTX binding in solubilized chicken optic lobe membranes at a concentration comparable to that in innervated skeletal muscle (Wang et al. 1978). This component from optic lobe shows high-affinity binding to iodinated α-BuTX with specific activities of 4000–6000 nmol/g protein. The component purified from "brain" (remainder of the brain after optic lobe removal) showed similar binding characteristics and specific activity. The optic lobe AChR, purified by α-BuTX-Sepharose affinity chromatography, sediments in sucrose gradients as a peak with a sedimentation coefficient of 10.1S – distinctly faster than muscle AChR centrifuged in parallel gradients (Conti-Tronconi et al. 1985). The molecular size of optic lobe AChR is significantly larger than muscle AChR, as shown by hydrodynamic determination with D_2O correction for bound detergent (data not shown).

Figure 1 shows a silver-stained SDS gel of purified optic lobe AChR. In different experiments five major components consistently appear, of apparent M_r 48K, 56K (doublet), 62K and 69K. This pattern differs from that previously reported (Norman et al. 1982; Betz and Pfeiffer 1984) and results from the use of an improved protocol for AChR isolation (Conti-Tronconi et al. 1985). What is the evidence that these polypeptides are homologous to peripheral AChR? We had previously shown that the 56K polypeptide could be affinity-labeled using bromoacetylcholine. Affinity labeling of intact receptor from optic lobe or brain specifically visualizes the 56K subunit (Fig. 2). Likewise, iodinated α-BuTX can be cross-linked to this subunit using dimethyl suberimidate. Thus, this subunit carries a high-affinity site for AChR and for toxin, as does the alpha subunit of the peripheral AChR.

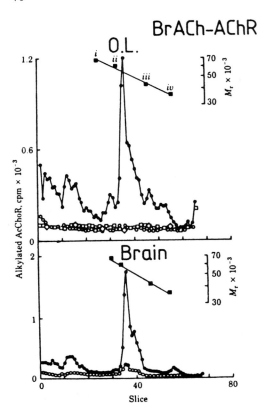

Fig. 2. Optic lobe or brain (see text) AChR was affinity-labeled with bromo[³H]acetylcholine and electrophoresed on a SDS gel which was then sliced and counted. *i-iv* represent the migration of molecular weight markers. (From Norman et al. 1982)

Additional evidence that at least some of the other polypeptides are components of the AChR was obtained by immunoprecipitation. We used a monoclonal antibody, 7B2, raised against chick muscle AChR which cross-reacts with the α-BuTX binding protein from chicken optic lobe (Mehraban et al. 1984). Optic lobe AChR was iodinated in vitro, immunoprecipitated with 7B2 and the precipitate analyzed on an SDS gel. The autoradiogram shows three bands are present, which correspond to the 48K, 56K and 69K bands seen upon SDS gel electrophoresis of non-iodinated receptor (Conti-Tronconi et al. 1985).

A 72,000-dalton polypeptide was also precipitated to some extent, but as it cannot be seen in the SDS gel of non-precipitated AChR, it is not at present considered to be part of the receptor. The 56K band again appears to be heterogeneous. Iodination clearly causes some breakdown of at least the 62K polypeptide — this is easily seen when the fluorographs of iodinated receptor are compared to silver- or Coomassie-stained gels of non-iodinated AChR. Since the 62K polypeptide cannot be immuno-precipitated (though possibly because of this degradation), there is no real evidence to support the contention that it forms part of a homologous AChR in optic lobe.

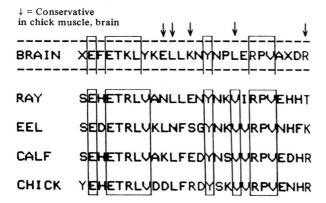

Fig. 3. The amino terminal amino acid sequence of the optic lobe 48K subunit is compared to that of the α-subunits of *Torpedo, Electrophorus,* calf and chick. *Boxes* enclose residues identical in all five AChRs and *arrows* represent conservative amino acid substitutions when chicken muscle and brain are compared. (From Conti-Tronconi et al. 1985)

Direct evidence for homology to muscle AChR has been obtained by amino-terminal microsequencing of isolated subunits. The four polypeptides visualised in optic lobe AChR were isolated by preparative SDS gel electrophoresis and aliquots were rerun to show purity. In at least three separate experiments using two different receptor preparations, the 48K polypeptide gave a single sequence. Amino terminal microsequence (ATAS) analysis of the other three isolated polypeptides gave no signal above background, indicating that they have blocked amino termini. This blockage occurs before subunit separation, since ATAS analysis of intact optic lobe preparations (containing all four subunits) gave a clear signal which corresponds to the sequence observed for the 48K polypeptide.

Comparison of the chemically determined amino terminal amino acid sequence of the 48K polypeptide with the known amino terminal sequences of chicken muscle AChR subunits shows that it is highly homologous to the chicken muscle alpha subunit (Fig. 3). The sequences can be aligned without introducing gaps and of the 26 residues available for comparison, 10 are identical. An additional five residues (shown by arrows in Fig. 3) represent chemically similar amino acid substitutions. The α-like nature of this polypeptide is further highlighted by the presence, in this brain protein, of stretches of amino acids diagnostic for the alpha subunit. These residues, glu-X-lys-leu at positions 4−7 (where X can be lys or arg but no other) and arg-pro-val at positions 20−22, occur in all known α-subunit sequences, but not in beta, gamma or delta.

In peripheral AChR, the α-subunit is known to be the subunit which is labeled by Br-ACh and binds α-BuTX. In the optic lobe AChR, we have shown that the α-like 48K subunit is not labeled, but the 56K polypeptide contains the site labeled by these reagents. Raftery and coworkers (personal communication) have noted that multiple ligand binding sites exist on *Torpedo* AChR and that Br-ACh can label other *Torpedo* subunits under different experimental conditions; thus it is possible that in the divergent CNS receptor that a different subunit is more easily labeled. To summarize, the isolated optic lobe AChR appears to be an oligomeric protein which shows structural similarities to, but is significantly different than the peripheral AChR: (1) the receptor is a larger complex, sedimenting at 10.1S, (2) four polypeptides of M_r 48, 56, 62 and 69K are consistently isolated, (3) one subunit shows distinct homology to all known α-subunits and (4) another subunit can be labeled with Br-ACh and cross-linked to α-BuTX.

7. Cloning Brain AChR Genes

Experiments currently in progress aim to isolate the gene encoding the 48K polypeptide. We used the cross-hybridization approach — a fragment encoding the transmembrane regions M1, M2 and M3 of the chicken muscle α-subunit was used to screen a λgt10 optic lobe cDNA library (Huynh et al. 1985; Watson and Jackson 1985) of 200,000 clones; four positively hybridizing plaques were detected. This is a frequency of 0.002%, approximately the same abundance with which α AChR sequences are present in innervated skeletal muscle mRNA and the λgt10 library prepared therefrom (see above). The concentration of α-BuTX binding sites in the two tissues is similar (Wang et al. 1978). Nucleotide sequence analysis of two of these clones shows that they appear to encode transmembrane and carboxy-terminal portions of a novel α-subunit homologous polypeptide (data not shown). Not surprisingly, they did not hybridize to short oligonucleotide probes derived from the ATAS sequence. We are currently testing the presumed tissue-specific expression of these clones.

In a second approach, a single long oligonucleotide presenting a "best-guess" 48-mer has been synthesized. These probes are designed to reflect the bias in codon usage for a given organism. Detection of homologous sequences in the genome tolerates a rather surprising degree of mismatch (Anderson and Kingston 1983; Jaye et al. 1983; Ullrich et al. 1984a,b). This probe is being used in hybridization experiments to a chicken genomic library. Cloning other components of the optic lobe AChR is likely to depend either upon sequencing free N-termini of internal regions of these polypeptides generated by limited proteolysis of intact subunits or the development of conformation-independent antibodies capable of detecting other subunits.

Acknowledgments. We would like to thank Drs. Brian Richards (Searle) and Michael Raftery (Caltech) for their continued interest in and support of the work described. The work at Caltech is supported by grants from the NIH and that at Imperial College is supported by grants from the MRC.

References

Anderson S, Kingston IB (1983) Isolation of a genomic clone for bovine pancreatic trypsin inhibitor by using a unique-sequence synthetic DNA probe. Proc Natl Acad Sci USA 80:6838–6842
Ballivet M, Nef P, Stalder R, Fulpius B (1983) Genomic sequences encoding the α-subunit of acetylcholine receptor are conserved during evolution. Cold Spring Harbor Symp Quant Biol 48:83–88

Beeson DMW, Barnard EA, Conti-Tronconi B, Dunn SMJ, Anderton T, Wilderspin AF, Bell LD, Jackson JF (1986) The chicken muscle acetylcholine receptor: subunit structure and the α-subunit cDNA cloning. J Biol Chem (in press)

Betz H, Pfeiffer F (1984) Monoclonal antibodies against the α-bungarotoxin-binding protein of chick optic lobe. J Neurosci 4:2095–2105

Conti-Tronconi BM, Raftery MA (1982) The nicotinic cholinergic receptor: correlation of molecular structure with functional properties. Annu Rev Biochem 51:491–530

Conti-Tronconi BM, Dunn SMJ, Barnard EA, Dolly JO, Lai FA, Ray N, Raftery MA (1985) Brain and muscle acetylcholine receptors are different but homologous proteins. Proc Natl Acad Sci USA 82:5208–5212

Dolly JO, Barnard EA (1984) Nicotinic acetylcholine receptors: an overview. Biochem Pharmacol 33:841–858

Greenberg ME, Ziff EB (1984) Stimulation of 3T3 cells induces transcription of the c-*fos* proto-oncogene. Nature 311:433–437

Huynh TV, Young RA, Davis RM (1985) Constructing and screening cDNA libraries in λgt10 and λgt11. In: Glover D (ed) DNA cloning: a practical approach, vol I. IRL, Oxford, p 49

Jacob MH, Berg DK (1983) The ultrastructural localization of α-bungarotoxin binding sites in relation to synapses on chick ciliary ganglion neurons. J Neurosci 3:260–271

Jayne M, de la Salle H, Schamber F, Balland A, Kohli V, Findeli A, Tolstoshev P, Lecocq (1983) Isolation of a human anti-haemophilic factor IX cDNA clone using a unique 52 base synthetic oligonucleotide probe deduced from the amino acid sequence of bovine factor IX. Nuclei Acids Res 11:2325–2335

Karlin A (1980) Molecular properties of nicotinic acetylcholine receptors. In: Cotman CW, Poste G, Nicolson GL (eds) The cell surface and neuronal function. Elsevier/North Holland, Amsterdam, p 191

Kistler J, Stroud RM, Klymkowsky MW, Lalancette RA (1982) Structure and function of an acetylcholine receptor. Biophys J 38:371–383

Marshall LM (1981) Synaptic localization of α-bungarotoxin binding which blocks nicotinic transmission at frog sympathetic neurons. Proc Natl Acad Sci USA 78:1948–1952

Mehraban F, Kemshead JT, Dolly JO (1984) Properties of monoclonal antibodies to nicotinic acetylcholine receptors from chick muscle. Eur J Biochem 138:53–61

Merlie JP, Isenberg KE, Russell SD, Sanes JR (1984) Denervation supersensitivity in skeletal muscle: analysis with a cloned cDNA probe. J Cell Biol 99:332–335

Morley BJ, Kemp GE (1981) Characterisation of a putative nicotinic acetylcholine receptor in mammalian brain. Brain Res Rev 3:81–104

Nef P, Mauron AS, Stalder C, Alliod C, Ballivet M (1984) Structure, linkage and sequence of the two genes encoding the delta and gamma subunits of the nicotinic acetylcholine receptor. Proc Natl Acad Sci USA 81:7975–7979

Noda M, Furutani Y, Takahashi H, Toyosato M, Tanabe T, Shimizu S, Kikyotani S, Kayano T, Hirose T, Inayama S, Numa S (1983) Cloning and sequence analysis of cell cDNA and human genomic DNA encoding α-subunit precursor of muscle acetylcholine receptor. Nature 305: 8181–823

Norman RI, Mehraban F, Barnard EA, Dolly JO (1982) Nicotinic acetylcholine receptor from chick optic lobe. Proc Natl Acad Sci USA 79:1321–1325

Oswald RE, Freeman JA (1981) Alpha-bungarotoxin binding and central nervous system nicotinic acetylcholine receptors. Neurosci 6:1–14

Popot J-L, Changeux J-P (1984) Nicotinic receptor of acetylcholine: structure of an oligomeric integral membrane protein. Phys Rev 64:1162–1239

Raftery MA, Junkapiller MW, Strader CD, Hood LE (1980) Acetylcholine receptor: complex of homologous subunits. Science 208:1454–1457

Sumikawa K, Houghton M, Smith JC, Bell L, Richards BM, Barnard EA (1982) The molecular cloning and characterisation of cDNA coding for the α subunit of the acetylcholine receptor. Nucleic Acids Res 10:5809–5822

Syapin PJ, Salvaterra PM, Engelhardt JK (1982) Neuronal-like features of TE671 cells: presence of a functional nicotinic cholinergic receptor. Brain Res 231:365–377

Takai T, Noda M, Furutani Y, Takahashi H, Notake M, Shimizu S, Kayano T, Tanabe T, Tanaka K, Hirose T, Inayama S, Numa S (1984) Primary structure of gamma subunit precursor of calf-muscle acetylcholine receptor deduced from the cDNA sequence. Eur J Biochem 143:109–115

Ullrich A, Coussens L, Hayflick JS, Dull TJ, Gray A, Tam AW, Lee J, Yarden Y, Libermann TA, Schlessinger J, Downward J, Mayes ELV, Whittle N, Waterfield MD, Seeburg PH (1984a) Human epidermal growth factor receptor cDNA sequence and aberrant expression of the amplified gene in A431 epidermoid carcinoma cells. Nature 309:418–425

Ullrich A, Berman CH, Dull TJ, Gray A, Lee JM (1984b) Isolation of the human insulin-like growth factor I gene using a single synthetic DNA probe. EMBO J 3:361–364

Wang GK, Molinaro S, Schmidt J (1978) Ligand responses of α-bungarotoxin binding sites from skeletal muscle and optic lobe of the chick. J Biol Chem 253:8507-8512

Watson CJ, Jackson JF (1985) An alternative procedure for the synthesis of double-stranded cDNA for cloning in phage and plasmid vectors. In: Glover D (ed) DNA cloning: a practical approach, vol I. IRL, Oxford, p 79

Regulation of Synapse-specific Genes

J.P. MERLIE and J.R. SANES[1]

In its distinctive form and specialized function the postsynaptic apparatus of the neuromuscular junction has many of the characteristics of an organelle; a tissue-specific one to be sure. Like other organelles, the junctional apparatus is formed and maintained by genetically programmed mechanisms which are modulated by environmental cues. For example, embryonic myotubes and denervated adult fibers assemble synaptic specializations under the influence of nerve terminals, and once innervated, a muscle will not easily form additional synapses. Thus, regulatory signals must pass between nerve and muscle to insure the formation and proper maintenance of the synapse. Recognition of the similarities between the synapse and other organelles has prompted us to consider the possibility that the genetic expression of components of the synapse is regulated by a common and synapse specific mechanism.

The neuromuscular junction is also highly specialized in its molecular composition, containing high concentrations of several cytoskeletal, membrane and extracellular matrix components that are virtually absent from extrasynaptic portions of the muscle fiber surface. The best studied of these synapse specific proteins is the acetylcholine receptor (AChR). AChRs are present throughout the membrane of embryonic myotubes, but become concentrated at synapses and are lost from extrasynaptic areas after synapses form. However, denervation or paralysis of adult muscle induces synthesis and insertion of new AChRs in extrasynaptic areas (Fig. 1). These alterations in AChR levels parallel the muscle fiber's ability to form new synapses, a parallel which extends, at least in part, to several other synapse specific molecules (Table 1). Therefore, it seems likely that the mechanisms which regulate the synthesis of synapse-specific molecules are, in fact, important components of the program which regulates the formation and maintenance of synapses.

In order to understand the intricacies of this program, we have begun studying the mechanisms of regulation of AChR levels in developing, normal adult and denervated adult muscle. Using cloned cDNA probes for mouse α (Merlie et al. 1983a) and δ (LaPolla et al. 1984) subunits, we have shown previously that AChR mRNA levels increase during differentiation of embryonic muscle cells in culture (Merlie et al. 1983b; and unpublished). In contrast, the levels detected in normal adult muscle are very low — 100-fold less than in the differentiated embryonic myotubes. Denervation

1 Departments of Pharmacology and of Anatomy and Neurobiology, Washington University, School of Medicine, St. Louis, MO 63110, USA

Molecular Aspects of Neurobiology
(ed. by Rita Levi Montalcini et al.)
© Springer-Verlag Berlin Heidelberg 1986

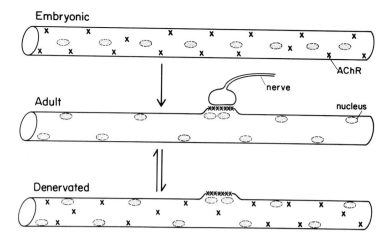

Fig. 1. AChRs are present throughout the membrane of embryonic myotubes. AChRs are lost extrasynaptically and become concentrated at the synapse as the muscle matures. Denervation leads to reappearance of extrasynaptic AChRs. Note that while nuclei are distributed along the muscle fiber, a few are directly beneath the postsynaptic membrane

of adult muscle results in a rapid 100-fold increase in AChR mRNA levels, an increase that slightly precedes the increase in AChR levels. The level of skeletal muscle actin mRNA changes little on denervation, emphasizing the specificity of the change in AChR mRNA (Merlie et al. 1984). These results suggest that the transcription and/or post-transcriptional processing of AChR mRNAs are subject to a dual control. The first is the activation of gene expression associated with terminal differentiation of myogenic cells. The second is the negative effect of nerve-induced muscle activity.

An important consequence of the hypothesis that activity suppresses transcription of AChR genes, is that one must then explain how high concentrations of AChR are maintained at the adult synapse. Since synaptic receptors turn over (Berg and Hall 1975; Salpeter and Harris 1983), they must be replaced by ongoing synthesis. One possibility is that synaptic receptors, which differ subtly from extrasynaptic and embryonic receptors (Hall et al. 1983), are encoded by a different set of genes. However, there is growing evidence, at least for α and δ subunits, that both synaptic and extrasynaptic AChRs are encoded by the same genes in the mouse (Merlie et al. 1983a; LaPolla et al. 1984; see also Noda et al. 1983; Klarsfeld et al. 1984; Nef et al. 1984; Shibahara et al. 1985). A second possibility is that receptors are synthesized uniformly along the length of the multinucleate fiber as a consequence of a basal level of subunit mRNA transcription. In this case, one might imagine that post translational steps, such as assembly of subunits or insertion into membrane, would be more efficient in synaptic areas. In fact, some post-translational regulation is detectable in tissue culture (Olson et al. 1983), the greater metabolic stability of synaptic than extrasynaptic AChR (Berg and Hall 1975) probably contributes to their concentration at synaptic sites. A third and, to us, particularly intriguing possibility is that AChR synthesis may be higher near to than far from synapses. The fact that muscle fibers are

Table 1. Synapse-specific molecules which may be coordinately regulated in muscle

	AChR (1)	N-CAM (2)	JS-1 (3)	AChE (4)	Cytoskeletal elements (5)
Concentrated in or near postsynaptic membrane	+	+	+	+	+
In extrasynaptic membrane in embryo	+	+		+	
Increased after denervation	+	+		+/−	+
Suppressed by activity/ increased by paralysis	+	+	+	−	
Increased by brain extract	+		+	+	

References: (1) Fambrough (1979); (2) Covault and Sanes (1985); (3) Sanes et al. (1984); (4) Massoulié and Bon (1982); (5) Bloch and Hall (1983); Chiu and Sanes (unpublished)

multinucleated raises the possibility that transcription of AChR mRNA might itself be differentially regulated along the length of the muscle: Adult muscle fibers typically have several hundred nuclei distributed along their length, but a few nuclei (3—5, or about 1% of the total) are invariably situated directly beneath the postsynaptic membrane. One might therefore imagine that synaptic and extrasynaptic nuclei could transcribe different sets of genes. In support of this possibility we have found recently that AChR mRNA is concentrated near synapses in adult muscle.

Our experiments have exploited the convenient anatomy of the mouse diaphragm. Most of the synapses and the great majority of the AChRs in this muscle are concentrated in its central third. Diaphragms were dissected into central, synapse-rich and distal, synapse-free portions and poly A+ mRNA was prepared from each. RNAs were fractionated on agarose gels, transferred to nitrocellulose and probed with ^{32}P-cDNAs specific for α (Merlie et al. 1983) and δ (Lapolla et al. 1984) subunits of mouse AChR and with a cDNA specific for mouse skeletal muscle actin (Caravatti et al. 1982). The relative abundance of mRNA in the synapse-rich and synapse-free samples was determined from these Northern blots as previously described (Merlie et al 1984).

Figure 2 shows that whereas actin mRNA was equally distributed between synapse-rich and free samples (ratio 1.1 ± 0.2 mean ± SEM in 6 experiments), α and δ subunit mRNAs were several fold more abundant (2.9 ± 0.5 fold, n = 6, for α subunit; 9 and 14 in 2 experiments on δ subunit) in synapse-rich than in synapse-free regions of the diaphragm. Although the precise distribution of AChR mRNAs and the processes by which they become preferentially concentrated near synapses remain to be elucidated, we have adopted the following as a working hypothesis: In the adult muscle fiber, AChR genes are preferentially transcribed in nuclei located closest to the synapse.

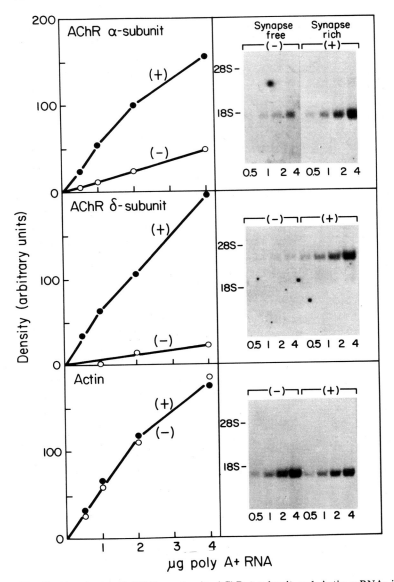

Fig. 2. Abundance of AChR α-subunit, AChR δ-subunit and Actin mRNAs in synapse-rich and synapse-free segments of diaphragm muscle. Graphs on *left* display results obtained by densitometry of autoradiographs of Northern blots, shown on *right*. The gels contained samples of 0.5–4 μg of total poly A+ RNA. Autoradiographs were exposed 7 d with intensifying screens for AChR subunit mRNA's and 12 h without intensifying screen for actin mRNA. (From Merlie and Sanes, to be published)

Synapse-associated nuclei, and the cytoplasm that surrounds them, are morphologically distinguishable from the nonsynaptic nuclei and cytoplasm (Couteaux 1973). Since only about 1% of all muscle fiber nuclei are synaptic, these nuclei might transcribe AChR mRNAs at the maximal rates characteristic of nuclei in denervated and embryonic muscle. How could transcription of AChR genes be maintained at a high level in synaptic nuclei while transcription from extrasynaptic nuclei was efficiently suppressed? Transcription at synaptic nuclei might be stimulated by the localized action of a trophic factor released by the motor neuron (see for example Buc-Caron et al. 1983). Alternatively, synaptic nuclei may escape the intracellular mediator of activity-linked down regulation, by virtue of their location in a unique region of the muscle cytoplasm.

A simple extension of this hypothesis is to postulate that AChR genes are members of a family of genes that are subject to similar transcriptional controls. As noted above, several proteins have already been described that are highly concentrated at synaptic sites on muscle fibers, and some of these are more widely distributed in embryonic muscle and/or induced to accumulate extrasynaptically by denervation of adult muscle (Table 1). We are currently attempting to assay the mRNAs that encode some of these proteins, to ask whether their levels vary in parallel with those of AChR subunit mRNAs.

In summary, our results raise the possibility that a small family of genes for synapse-specific proteins may be coordinately regulated by mechanisms which contribute importantly to synapse formation. While these genes may be turned on along with a larger group of muscle-specific genes during myogenesis, their subsequent regulation differs: Expression of the synapse-specific family is, in addition, suppressed by electrical activity. This simple model predicts that genes of the synaptic family might be associated with at least two types of homologous regulatory sequences: one involved in developmental expression during myogenesis, and a second involved in activity-linked suppression. A third regulatory system might induce transcription of these genes in synaptic nuclei, and/or render synaptic nuclei immune to the repressive effects of activity. Therefore, it will be important to search for homologies in the regulatory sequences associated with genes of members of this family.

References

Berg DK, Hall ZW (1975) Loss of α-bungarotoxin from junctional and extrajunctional acetylcholine receptors in rat diaphragm *in vivo* and organ culture. J Physiol (Lond) 252:771–789

Bloch RJ, Hall ZW (1983) Cytoskeletal components of the vertebrate neuromusclular junction: Vinculin, α-actinin, and filamin. J Cell Biol 97:217–223

Buc-Caron MH, Nystrom P, Fischbach GD (1983) Induction of acetylcholine receptor synthesis and aggregation: partial purification of low-molecular-weight activity. Dev Biol 95:378–386

Caravatti M, Minty A, Robert B, Montarras D, Weydert A, Cohen A, Daubas P, Buchingham M (1982) Regulation of muscle gene expression: the accumulation of messenger RNA's coding for muscle-specific proteins during myogenesis in a mouse cell line. J Mol Biol 160:59–76

Couteaux R (1973) Motor end plate structure: In: Bourne GH (ed) The structure and function of muscle, vol II. Academic, New York, p 483

Covault J, Sanes JR (1985) Neural cell adhesion molecule (N-CAM) accumulates in denervated and paralyzed skeletal muscles. Proc Natl Acad Sci USA 82:4544–4548

Fambrough DM (1979) Control of acetylcholine receptors in skeletal muscle. Physiol Rev 59:165–226

Hall ZW, Roizin MP, Gu Y, Gorin PD (1983) A developmental change in the immunological properties of the acetylcholine receptors at the rat neuromuscular junction. Cold Spring Harbor Symp Quant Biol 40:263–274

Klarsfeld A, Devillers-Thiéry A, Giraudat J, Changeux J-P (1984) A single gene codes for the nicotinic acetylcholine receptor α-subunit in *Torpedo marmorata:* Structural and developmental implications. EMBO J 3:35–41

LaPolla RJ, Mixter Mayne K, Davidson N (1984) Isolation and characterization of a cDNA clone for the complete protein coding region of the δ subunit of the mouse acetylcholine receptor. Proc Natl Acad Sci USA 81:7970–7974

Massoulié J, Bon S (1982) The molecular forms of cholinesterase and acetylcholinesterase in vertebrates. Annu Rev Neurosci 5:57–106

Merlie JP, Sanes JR (to be published) Acetylcholine receptor mRNA is concentrated in synaptic regions of adult muscle fibres

Merli JP, Sebbane R, Gardner S, Lindstrom J (1983a) cDNA clone for the α subunit of the acetylcholine receptor from the mouse muscle cell line BC3H-1. Proc Natl Acad Sci USA 80:3845–3849

Merlie JP, Sebbane R, Gardner S, Olson E, Lindstrom J (1983b) The regulation of acetylcholine receptor expression in mammalian muscle. Cold Spring Harbor Symp Quant Biol 48:135–145

Merlie JP, Isenberg K, Russell S, Sanes JR (1984) Denervation supersensitivity in skeletal muscle: analysis with a cloned cDNA probe. J Cell Biol 99:332–335

Nef P, Mauron A, Stalder R, Alliod C, Ballivet M (1984) Structure, linkage, and sequence of the two genes encoding the δ and γ subunits of the nicotinic acetylcholine receptor. Proc Natl Acad Sci USA 81:7975:7979

Noda M, Furutani Y, Takahashi H, Toyosato M, Tanabe T, Shimizu S, Kikyotani S, Kayano T, Hirose T, Inayama S, Numa S (1983) Cloning and sequence analysis of calf cDNA and human genomic DNA encoding α-subunit precursor of muscle acetylcholine receptor. Nature 305:818–823

Olson EN, Glaser L, Merlie JP, Sebbane R, Lindstrom J (1983) Regulation of surface expression of acetylcholine receptors in response to serum and cell growth in the BC3H-1 mouse cell line. J Biol Chem 258:13946–13953

Salpeter MM, Harris RJ (1983) Distribution and turnover rate of acetylcholine receptors throughout the junction folds at a vertebrate neuromuscular junction. J Cell Biol 96:1791–1785

Sanes JR, Feldman DH, Cheney JM, Lawrence JC Jr (1984) Brain extract induces synaptic characteristics in the basal lamina of cultured myotubes. J Neurosci 4:464–473

Shibahara S, Kubo T, Perski HS, Takahashi H, Noda M, Numa S (1985) Cloning and sequence analysis of human genomic DNA encoding γ subunit precursor of muscle acetylcholine receptor. Eur J Biochem 146:15–22

Asymmetrical Distribution of Membrane-bound Cytoskeleton Proteins at the Innervated and Non-innervated Membrane Domains in Torpedo Electrocytes

C. KORDELI[1], J. CARTAUD[1], H.O. NGHIÊM[2], and J.P. CHANGEUX[2]

1. Introduction

Cell polarity evidenced in many cells on behavioral, functional or structural bases is generally accompanied by a cytoskeleton asymmetry.

The fish electric organ unitary cell, the electrocyte, is a good example of a differentiated cell that elaborated and maintained two functionally specialized domains of the plasma membrane. The innervated and non-innervated membranes are engaged respectively in acetylcholine-mediated chemical excitability or regeneration of the electrochemical gradient. Associated with these functions, the two domains of the plasma membrane accumulated specific molecular species, the acetylcholine receptor (AChR) and the Na^+K^+ ATPase.

Excitable membrane fragments purified from adult *T. marmorata* electric tissue contain, in addition to the AChR polypeptides, a major extrinsic component of Mr 43,000 dalton (43 kd) probably engaged in the immobilization of the membrane-bound receptors (Cartaud et al. 1981; Neubig et al. 1979).

In this work, we established, using immunocytochemical methods, that topographical relationships between each of the electrocyte membrane domains and specific cytoskeletal components exist, leading to an anisotropic organization of the cortex of the cell.

2. Membrane-cytoskeleton Interactions at the Innervated Face of T. marmorata Electrocyte

Immunofluorescence experiments demonstrated that both the AChR and the 43 kd protein were localized on the innervated face of the cell (Fig. 1). At the electron microscope level, the two components were observed uniquely on the postsynaptic membrane. The 43 kd protein appeared strictly associated with the cytoplasmic sur-

[1] Microscopie Electronique, Institut J. Monod, CNRS, Université Paris VII, 2 Place Jussieu, 75005, Paris, France
[2] Neurobiologie Moléculaire, Institut Pasteur, 25 Rue du Dr. Roux, 75015 Paris, France

Molecular Aspects of Neurobiology
(ed. by Rita Levi Montalcini et al.)
© Springer-Verlag Berlin Heidelberg 1986

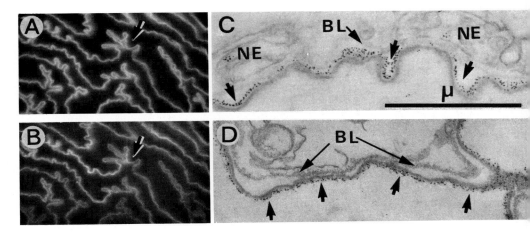

Fig. 1A–D. Immunocytochemical localization of AChR and 43 kd proteins in cryostat sections of *T. marmorata* electric tissue. **A, B** show that same section treated in **A** with rhodamine-α-bungaro-toxin, and in **B** with anti-43 kd monoclonal antibody (m ab) revealed by a second fluorescein-coupled antibody. Note that AChR and 43 kd molecules strictly codistribute (× 300). **C, D** Electron micrographs show the localization of AChR and 43 kd by the immunogold technique. Note that the 43 kd protein is associated with the cytoplasmic face of the postsynaptic membrane. *BL* basal lamina; *NE* nerve ending

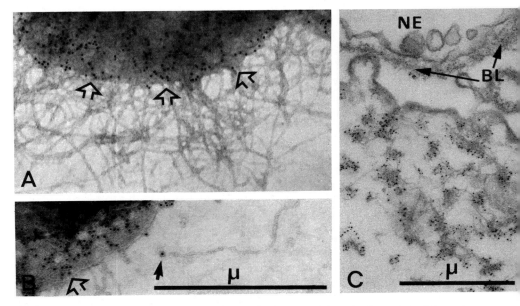

Fig. 2A–C. Membrane-cytoskeleton association at the innervated face. **A** Ghost derived from the innervated membrane labeled with the anti-43 kd m ab is visualized by negative staining. A dense network of intermediate-sized filaments is attached to the labeled membrane surface (*arrows*). **B** Detail showing an end-on labeling of an individual filament detached from the 43 kd-labeled membrane. **C** Membrane ghost after labeling with an anti-desmine antibody

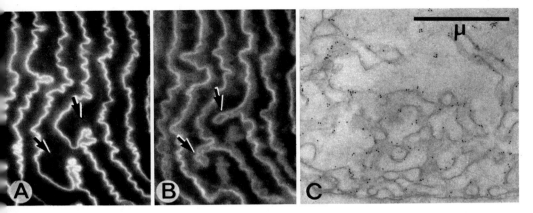

Fig. 3A–C. Subcellular distribution of ankyrin in *Torpedo* sections **A, B** show the same section treated in **A** with rhodamine-α-bungarotoxin, and in **B** with anti-ankyrin affinity purified antibody. The antibody labeling does not codistribute with toxin-labeled AChR but rather occurs on the opposite, non-innervated face of the electrocytes (× 300). **C** Electron micrograph shows a membrane sheet derived for the non-innervated face of the cell, labeled with the anti-ankyrin antibody

face of the AChR-rich domains of the membrane (Nghiêm et al. 1983; Sealock et al. 1984). The non-innervated membrane was never labeled with the anti-43 kd antibody.

On the other hand, intermediate-sized filaments identified by their EM appearance form the bulk of the transcellular skeleton of the electrocyte and terminate on both surfaces of the cell. These filaments were decorated with an anti-desmin antibody (Fig. 2). Interestingly, ends of detached filaments were sometimes labeled with the anti-43 kd antibody (Fig. 2), raising the possibility that the AChR molecules are anchored to the underlying intermediate filament meshwork via the 43 kd protein (Cartaud et al. 1983).

Despite an important G actin pool dispersed within the cytoplasm, no actin filaments were identified yet, in ʼarticular on the innervated membrane.

3. Membrane-cytoskeleton Interaction at the Non-innervated Membrane

The non-innervated side of the electrocyte is characterized by numerous tubular infoldings of the plasma membrane that contain the Na^+K^+ ATPase. In the present study we showed that two proteins, previously identified as major components of the cortical skeleton on the red blood cell, spectrin (or fodrin) and ankyrin (Branton et al. 1981) are present on the non-innervated membrane (Fig. 3). In the erythrocytes, small actin polymers are associated to the membrane skeleton via an interaction with spectrin (Branton et al. 1981). A similar form of actin was revealed with rhodamine-phalloidin on the non-innervated membrane.

In conclusion, we have identified within the electrocyte an anisotropical arrangement of some cytoskeletal proteins that codistribute respectively with the innervated, AChR-rich and the non-innervated, ATPase-rich domains of the plasma membrane. This organization brings possible biochemical bases for the maintenance or even the origin of the electrocyte polarity.

Acknowledgments. We thank Drs. D. Paulin, A.L. Pradel, S. Tzartos for gifts of antibodies and Dr. M. Vigny for a gift of rhodamine-α-bungarotoxin.

References

Branton D, Cohen CM, Tyler J (1981) Interaction of cytoskeletal proteins on the human erythrocyte membrane. Cell 24:24—32

Cartaud J, Sobel A, Rousselet A, Devaux PF, Changeux JP (1981) Consequence of alkaline treatment for the ultrastructure of the acetylcholine-receptor-rich membranes from *Torpedo marmorata* electric organ. J Cell Biol 90:418—426

Cartaud J, Kordeli C, Nghiêm HO, Changeux JP (1983) La protéine v_1 de 43,000 dalton: pièce intermédiaire assurant l'ancrage du recepteur cholinergique au cytosquelette sous-neural? CR Acad Sci Paris 297:285—289

Neubig RR, Krodel EK, Boyd ND, Cohen JB (1979) Acetylcholine and local anesthetic binding to *Torpedo* nicotinic postsynaptic membrane after removal of non receptor peptides. Proc Natl Acad Sci USA 76:690—694

Nghiêm HO, Cartaud J, Dubreuil C, Kordeli C, Buttin G, Changeux JP (1983) Production and characterization of a monoclonal antibody directed against the 43,000 dalton v_1, polypeptide from *T. marmorata* electric organ. Proc Natl Acad Sci USA 80:6403—6407

Sealock R, Wray BE, Froehner S (1984) Ultrastructural localization of the Mr 43,000 protein and the acetylcholine receptor in Torpedo postsynaptic membranes using monoclonal antibodies. J Cell Biol 98:2239—2244

In Search of the Binding Site of the Nicotinic Acetylcholine Receptor

J.M. GERSHONI, D. NEUMANN, and S. FUCHS[1]

It is well accepted that the ligand-binding site of the nicotinic acetylcholine receptor (AChR) is harbored, at least in part, in the receptor α-subunit (Popot and Changeux 1984; Conti-Tronconi and Raftery 1982; Karlin 1983). Probing this site with α-bungarotoxin (BTX) is especially convenient due to its high affinity for it (10^{-11} M). The fact that the affinity alkylating analogue of ACh, i.e. maleimido-benzyl trimethyl ammonium bromide (MBTA), can irreversibly block both toxin and ACh binding to AChR, has been taken as proof that indeed the toxin binding site is either in close proximity to, or equal with the cholinergic binding site (Karlin 1983). Moreover, as MBTA binds via a maleimido moiety, a Cys residue should be present no more than 1 nm away from the actual site (Karlin 1983). Thus, much effort has been devoted towards localizing the ligand binding site on the AChR α-subunit and identifying the alkylated Cys residue.

With the advent of recombinant DNA cloning, the complete amino acid sequence of the AChR has been postulated (Noda et al. 1982, 1983; Claudio et al. 1983). The sequence data has been the basis of quite a few models which hypothesize the orientation of the α-subunit as it traverses the lipid bilayer (reviewed in Popot and Changeux 1984). Furthermore, a number of laboratories have promoted models of the ligand binding site which are fitted to selected amino acid sequences of the α-subunit (e.g. Smart et al. 1984). In this presentation we describe experimental data from which we conclude that the cholinergic binding site resides C-terminal to Asp 152 and is in close proximity to or contiguous with Cys 192.

By way of protein blotting it can be shown that BTX binds to isolated immobilized α-subunit (Gershoni et al. 1983). In this procedure, AChR is separated into its constituents by polyacrylamide gel electrophoresis. The resolved subunits are then electrophoretically transferred to an immobilizing matrix which is subsequently probed with radioactive BTX. Both glycosylated and deglycosylated α-subunit bind BTX. The binding is competed with antagonists, e.g. tubocurarine and can be blocked with MBTA. BTX overlays of blotted proteolytic digests of the α-subunit reveal that fragments as small as 8K can still retain binding activity (Wilson et al. 1984).

1 Departments of Biophysics and Chemical Immunology, Weizmann Institute of Science, Rehovot, Israel

Molecular Aspects of Neurobiology
(ed. by Rita Levi Montalcini et al.)
© Springer-Verlag Berlin Heidelberg 1986

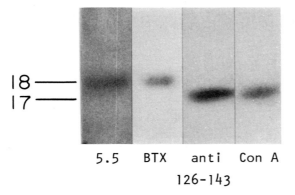

18 ——
17 ——

5.5   BTX   anti   Con A

126-143

Fig. 1. Blot analysis of *S. aureus* V8 proteolysed α-subunit. Protein blots of proteolysed α-subunit of AChR were prepared as previously described (Wilson et al. 1984). The blots were probed with the cholinergic-site specific monoclonal antibody *5.5, BTX,* antipeptide *126–143* antibody or concanavalin *A* as indicated

In order to pinpoint the precise amino acid sequence responsible for ligand binding, probes, highly specific for selected amino acid sequences of the α-subunit were prepared. This was achieved by constructing synthetic peptides corresponding to two putative cholinergic binding sites, i.e. residues 1–20 (Smythies 1980) and 126–143 (Noda et al. 1982). Polyclonal antibodies were prepared in rabbits against the synthetic peptides and were found to associate specifically to the α-subunit of AChR (Neumann et al. 1984, 1985). Moreover, in probing blots of proteolysed α-subunit it was found that distinct peptide fragments could be demonstrated to bind the antibodies with no cross-reaction between them (Neumann et al. 1985).

As can be seen in Fig. 1, when α-subunit is proteolysed with *S. aureus* V8 protease only one peptide fragment, 18K, binds BTX. This fragment has previously been shown to bind MBTA as well (Gullick et al. 1981; Wilson et al. 1984). Moreover, it also binds the binding site specific monoclonal antibody 5.5 (Mochly-Rosen and Fuchs 1982). In contrast to this, a 17K fragment can be identified with the antipeptide 126–143 antibody. This fragment is also N-glycosylated as is demonstrated by its concanavalin A binding (Fig. 1) and its sensitivity to endoglycosidase H treatment (Neurmann et al. 1985). This demonstrates the presence of Asn 141, the only asparagine residue of the α-subunit that can be N-glycosylated.

Thus, by *S. aureus* V8 proteolysis, we have generated a 18K fragment which as we have shown lacks the N-terminal sequence 1–20, as well as the peptide sequence 126–143 and Asn 141 yet still binds BTX. This BTX binding is MBTA sensitive, indicative of the presence of alkylated Cys residues (Wilson et al. 1984). As Cys 128 and 142 are not present in the 18K fragment and thus are not required for BTX binding, our results not only support the recent paper of Kao et al. (1984) claiming that Cys 192 is MBTA alkylated, but demonstrate that the toxin binding site is physically close to this residue.

Acknowledgments. This work was supported by grants from the Muscular Dystrophy Association of America, the Los Angeles Chapter of the Myasthenia Gravis Foundation, the United States-Israel Binational Science Foundation (BSF) and the Batsheva de Rothschild Foundation for the Advancement of Science.

References

Claudio T, Ballivet M, Patrick J, Heinemann S (1983) Proc Natl Acad Sci USA 80:1111–1115

Conti-Tronconi BM, Raftery MA (1982) Annu Rev Biochem 51:491–530

Gershoni JM, Hawrot E, Lentz TL (1983) Proc Natl Acad Sci USA 80:4973–4977

Gullick WJ, Tzartos S, Lindstrom J (1981) Biochemistry 20:2178–2189

Kao PN, Dwork AJ, Kaldany RJ, Silver ML, Wideman J, Stein S, Karlin A (1984) J Biol Chem 259: 11662–11665

Karlin A (1983) Neurosci Commun 3:111–123

Mochly-Rosen D, Fuchs S (1982) Biochemistry 20:5920–5924

Neumann D, Fridkin M, Fuchs S (1984) Biochem Biophys Res Commun 121:673–679

Neumann D, Gershoni JM, Fridkin M, Fuchs S (1985) Proc Natl Acad Sci USA (in press)

Noda M et al. (1982) Nature 299:793–797

Noda M et al. (1983) Nature 301:251–255

Popot J-L, Changeux J-P (1984) Physiol Rev 6:1162–1239

Smart L, Meyers H-W, Hilgenfeld R, Saenger W, Maelicke A (1984) FEBS Lett 178:64–68

Smythies JR (1980) Med Hypotheses 6:948–950

Wilson PT, Gershoni JM, Hawrot E, Lentz TL (1984) Proc Natl Acad Sci USA 81:2553–2557

Identification of Acetylcholine Receptors from the Central Nervous System of Insects

H. BREER[1]

The identification of the peripheral acetylcholine receptor (AChR) of vertebrates was greatly facilitated by employing α-toxins, notably α-bungarotoxin (α-BGTX). Although binding sites for α-BGTX have also been found in brain tissue, it is presently highly controversial whether these binding sites in the nervous tissue represent really functional receptors (Morley and Kemp 1981). In the central nervous system of insects, acetylcholine has been shown to be the major excitatory transmitter and several studies have recently demonstrated a very high concentration of specific binding sites for α-BGTX with a distinct nicotinic pharmacology (Breer 1981). For insect nervous tissue there is clear electrophysiological evidences that α-BGTX blocks the function of post-synaptic nicotinic receptors and the pharmacological data can be directly related to the binding data (Sattelle et al. 1983), suggesting that in insect nervous tissue the toxin binding sites represent acetylcholine receptors. Thus insect ganglia seemed to be a suitable tissue for characterizing the nicotinic acetylcholine receptor of nerve cells, which ultimately would allow to compare its molecular properties with the well-characterized receptor of muscle cells and electrocytes.

The nicotine acetylcholine receptor as probed by α-BGTX binding has been isolated from detergent solubilized neuronal membrane preparation of *Locusta migratoria* using centrifugation and chromatographical techniques and exists as a homogeneous protein species, when isolated under conditions designed to minimize protolytic degradation: it gives a single peak by centrifugation on sucrose gradient (10 S) and migrates as a single band on PAGE under nondenaturing conditions (M_r 250–300.000) as well as on SDS-PAGE (M_r 65.000), suggesting that the neuronal ACh represents an oligomeric complex of four very similar polypeptides (Breer et al. 1985). The identification of this protein as AChR is based on its saturable binding of α-BGTX specifically inhibited by nicotinic ligands (Breer et al. 1984), furthermore the purified AChR-polypeptides showed immunological cross-reactivity with a monoclonal anti(*Torpedo*-AChR)-antibody in immunoblots. In immunohistochemical studies using monospecific rabbit anti(locust-AChR)-antiserum, the immunoreactive sites were localized in specific areas of the neuropile, which are supposed to contain cholinergic synapses (Breer et al. 1985).

To ultimately prove, however, that the isolated polypeptides represent functional receptor molecules and not only ligand binding constituents it was necessary to recon-

---

1 University Osnabrück, Department of Zoophysiology, D–4500 Osnabrück, F.R.G.

Molecular Aspects of Neurobiology
(ed. by Rita Levi Montalcini et al.)
© Springer-Verlag Berlin Heidelberg 1986

stitute the protein in artificial lipid membranes. In collaboration with Dr. Hanke we have recently succeeded in reconstituting the purified receptor protein from insect nervous tissue into virtually solvent free planar lipid bilayers. Proteoliposomes containing the purified receptor protein were fused with bilayers to incorporate the AChR-receptor. Without any agonist present there was no ion channel fluctuation, however, when agonists were added, channels with conductance of about 75 pS and with a mean lifetime of about 10 ms appeared. Besides a larger conductance, the insect receptor showed about the same behavior as vertebrate peripheral receptors: elevated agonist concentrations increased the probability of a channel to be in the open state, the lifetimes of the open state become longer, but the conductance of the channel was always identical independent of the type and concentration of agonists (Hanke and Breer 1986). The receptor channel did not show any significant selectivity for sodium over potassium, but seems to be impermeable for chloride and appeared to behave ohmically over a range of voltage. These results demonstrated that the purified toxin binding protein from insect nervous tissue represents a functional transmitter receptor. Thus the AChR of insect appears to be an oligomeric membrane protein composed of four identical subunits (M_r 65.000) and it is thus significantly different from the heterooligomeric receptor of muscle cells and electrocytes.

The homooligomeric structure of the insect receptor is of particular interest in view of the receptor evolution. Based on immunological data and amino acid sequence homology of the four different polypeptides forming the vertebrate receptor, it has been suggested that the genes coding for the subunits of the receptor protein must have originated from a common ancestral gene via duplication (Raftery et al. 1980); the ancestral AChR-receptor is supposed to have been a homooligomeric complex from which the recent heterooligomeric receptors have evolved. Whether the homo-oligomeric receptor from insects can be considered as a representative of an ancient form is unclear, yet. However, the elucidation of its primary structure by cloning and sequencing the coding nucleic acids will show if there are any significant structural similarities between the insect and vertebrate receptor and may shed some new light on the molecular evolution of the acetylcholine receptor. As a first approach, the nervous tissue of locusts was probed for receptor-specific mRNA using the *Xenopus* oocytes as an assay system. The oocytes express microinjected mRNA with efficiency and perform all the posttranslational modification and even incorporate receptor proteins in the plasma membrane. Poly A^+-RNA isolated from the ganglia of young insects and microinjected into *Xenopus* oocytes induced the synthesis of α-bungaro-toxin binding proteins (Breer and Benke 1985). The binding sites showed about the same affinity and pharmacology of toxin binding as receptors in neuronal membranes. In order to identify the newly synthesized binding protein oocytes were incubated with radiolabeled amino acids and the protein immunprecipitated with monospecific antibodies. Autoradiographs of the electrophoresis gels showed only one labeled band at position of about 65 kd, showing that the oocytes had synthesized and processed the insect receptor polypeptides to its native size. To clarify whether the binding proteins in oocytes represent functional receptors ion flux studies were performed. The results demonstrated that in oocytes microinjected with poly A^+-RNA from insect after 1—2 days influx of ^{86}Rb could specifically be induced by cholinergic agonists; an effect never seen in non-injected oocytes and completely blocked by antagonists like d-tubocurarine. Thus it appears that functional acetylcholine receptors are produced in *Xenopus* oocytes after microinjection of mRNA from insect nervous system.

References

Breer H (1981) Properties of putative nicotinic and muscarinic cholinergic receptors in the central nervous system of *Locusta migratoria*. Neurochem Int 3:43–52

Breer H, Benke D (1985) Naturwissenschaften 72:213–214

Breer H, Kleene R, Benke D (1984) Isolation of a putative nicotinic receptor from the central nervous system of *Locusta migratoria*. Neurosci Lett 46:323–328

Breer H, Kleene R, Hinz G (1985) Molecular forms and subunit structure of the acetylcholine receptor in the central nervous system of insects. J Neurosci 5:3386–3392

Hanke W, Breer H (1986) Purified acetylcholine receptor protein from central nervous system of *Locusta migratoria* forms functional agonist activated ion channels in planar lipid bilayers. Nature (in press)

Morley BJ, Kemp GE (1981) Characterization of a putative nicotinic acetylcholine receptor in mammalian brain. Brain Res Rev 3:81–104

Raftery MA, Hunkapiller MW, Strader CD, Hood LE (1980) Acetylcholine receptor: complex of homologous subunits. Science 208:1454–1457

Sattelle DB, Harrow ID, Hue B, Pelhate M, Gepner JI, Hall LM (1983) α-bungarotoxin blocks excitatory synaptic transmission between cercal sensory neurons and giants interneurone 2 of the cockkroach *Periplaneta americana*. J Exp Biol 107:473–489

The GABA/Benzodiazepine Receptor Complex: Function, Structure and Location

H. MÖHLER, P. SCHOCH, and J.G. RICHARDS[1]

1. GABAergic Neurotransmission

In mammalian CNS, GABAergic synaptic transmission (GABA = γ-aminobutyric acid) is fundamental to inhibitory feedback and feedforward circuits of projecting neurons and local interneurons. Up to 30% of all synapses in the brain are thought to be GABA-ergic. The synaptic inhibitory action of GABA is due to the opening of GABA-gated chloride channels, which in turn leads to an increase in the chloride conductance of the subsynaptic membrane. Most frequently, the chloride flux is directed inward, leading to a hyperpolarizing inhibitory postsynaptic potential. In recent years, studies of the GABAergic inhibitory synaptic transmission have unraveled a molecular mechanism by which anxiety, vigilance, muscle tension and the occurrence of convulsions can be regulated.

2. Regulation of GABAergic Neurotransmission

The kinetics of the GABA gated chloride channel can be altered by drugs, notably by ligands of the benzodiazepine receptor (BZR). This receptor was originally identified as the target structure for benzodiazepines (Möhler and Okada 1977; Squires and Braestrup 1977), a group of drugs with wide therapeutic application as anxiolytics, hypnotics, muscle relaxants and anticonvulsants [Diazepam (Valium) as main representative]. Most, if not all, BZR are part or the GABA receptor complex where they serve as modulatory unit. In the presence of tranquillizing benzodiazepines the GABA-induced bursts of chloride channel opening are prolonged compared to those in the absence of the drug. This increase in the efficiency of GABAergic synaptic transmission produces the main therapeutic effects of the tranquillizing benzodiazepines (Table 1) (Haefely and Polc 1985).

   In recent years, novel BZR ligands were found by which the efficiency of GABA-ergic synaptic transmission was reduced. Correspondingly, these compounds show

1 Pharmaceutical Research Department, F. Hoffmann-La Roche & Co., Ltd., CH–4002 Basel, Switzerland

Table 1. Modulation of CNS functions by two types of benzodiazepine receptor (BZR) ligands

Agonists		Inverse agonists
−	Anxiety	+
−	Muscle tension	+
−	Convulsions	+
−	Vigilance	+

Agonists are those BZR ligands which enhance GABAergic synaptic transmission; inverse agonists reduce GABAergic transmission.
− indicates decrease of symptoms, + increase of symptoms

pharmacological effects opposite to those of BZR agonists. They can induce anxiety
attacks, increase muscle tension, precipitate convulsions and increase vigilance (Table 1).

The effects of both types of BZR ligands are mediated via the same binding domain
on the BZR. This could be clearly demonstrated in competition experiments with the
selective antagonist Ro 15-1788. By competitive interaction the effects of both types
of BZR ligands could be antagonized by Ro 15-1788 (Haefely 1985). A structural and
morphological analysis of the GABA receptor complex should provide a more detailed
understanding of the regulatory events at the receptor level.

3. Structure of the GABA Receptor Complex

The GABA receptor complex comprises three functional entities: the GABA receptor,
its associated chloride channel and the benzodiazepine receptor. Constituent proteins
of the GABA receptor complex were identified by photoaffinity labeling with photo-
reactive benzodiazepines (Möhler et al. 1980), by radiation inactivation (Chang and
Barnard 1982), by affinity purification of the receptor (Sigel and Barnard 1983;
Schoch et al. 1984) and by immunoreaction with monoclonal antibodies (Häring et al.
1985). These studies resulted in a largely uniform picture of the receptor-structure
(Möhler et al. 1985; Fig. 1). The receptor contains a 50 kd protein (α-subunit) and a
55 kd protein (β-subunit) as shown unequivocally by immunological studies. These
proteins are assumed to contain three types of binding sites: those for benzodiazepines,
for GABA (high and low affinity sites) and probably also for the convulsant TBPS
(t-butylbicyclophosphorothionate), which binds to a site affecting the chloride channel. The receptor is a glycoprotein which probably protrudes on the outer cell surface
as indicated by partial proteolytic digestion.

Comparison of the molecular weight of the subunits and the native receptor indi-
cates a tetrameric $\alpha_2\beta_2$ subunit arrangement. While the α and β subunits have a molecular weight of 50 kd and 55 kd, respectively, the target size for benzodiazepine and
GABA binding sites in membranes was 220 kd. Furthermore, a tetrameric model was
indicated by photoaffinity labeling experiments in which photoreaction to one benzo-

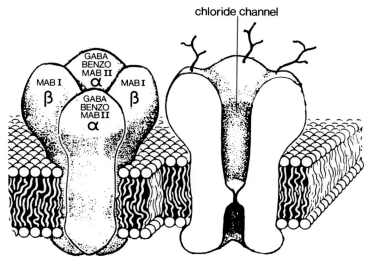

Fig. 1. Working hypothesis for a model of the GABA receptor complex (Möhler et al. 1985). α and β indicate the 50 kd and 55 kd subunits, respectively. *Benzo* indicates benzodiazepine binding sites identified by photolabeling. *GABA* indicates GABA binding sites identified by photolabeling. *MAB I, II* indicate epitopes recognized by subunit specific monoclonal antibodies. *Branched lines* are carbohydrate residues

diazepine binding site in the membrane allosterically blocked three additional sites. It is conceivable that the $\alpha_2\beta_2$ tetramer contains not only all the known binding sites of the receptor complex but also forms the chloride channel.

There is only limited information available which allows an allocation of the various ligand-binding sites to certain receptor domains. Binding sites for benzodiazepines are clearly located on the α-subunit. Conceivably, they might also occur on the β-subunit, although in a state which is generally not photolabeled. Electrophysiologically, two GABA sites were postulated per GABA receptor to gate the chloride channel. GABA sites were attributed biochemically to the α-subunit, although the possible presence of non-photolabeled GABA sites on the β-subunit cannot be excluded. The location of the TBPS binding sites is yet unknown. Binding sites may well occur in subunit interfaces.

The present working hypothesis may have to be modified in the future. There is experimental evidence from our group for the copurification of a protein in addition to the α- and β-subunit. Also, the TBPS binding site may include additional protein components. A final clarification of the protein composition of the GABA receptor complex is expected from reconstitution experiments. Reconstitution of the purified receptor in lipid bilayers has been achieved, as tested by radioligand binding (Schoch et al. 1984) but chloride flux measurements have not yet been accomplished.

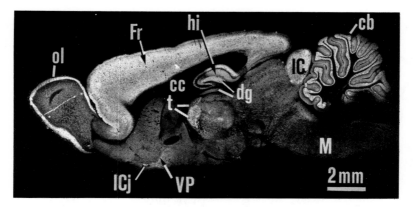

Fig. 2. Immunohistochemical localization of antigenic sites in a parasagittal section of rat brain using a monoclonal antibody (bd-17) raised against the GABA receptor complex (Schoch et al. 1985).
Abbreviations: *cb* cerebellum; *cc* corpus callosum; *Fr* frontal cerebral cortex; *dg* dentate gyrus; *hi* hippocampus; *ICj* islands of Calleja; *IC* inferior colliculus; *M* medulla; *ol* olfactory bulb; *t* thalamus; *VP* ventral pallidum

4. Location of the GABA Receptor Complex

The morphological analysis of the localization of the GABA receptor complex was in agreement with the role of the GABA receptor complex in synaptic transmission.

The receptor complex is exclusively localized in synaptic contacts. This was demonstrated by electronmicroscopic autoradiography after irreversible labeling of the receptor (Möhler et al. 1981) and by electronmicroscopic immunocytochemistry (Möhler et al. 1985). At least some of these synapses were identified as GABAergic as shown by staining the same slices with antiserum to glutamic acid decarboxylase, the marker enzyme of GABA neurons (Möhler et al. 1981). The receptor is clearly located on the postsynaptic membrane as shown immunocytochemically (Möhler et al. 1985). Immunoreactivity was also detected on the presynaptic membrane of the same synapses, suggesting that related GABA receptors, presumably autoreceptors, exist on GABA terminals. However, an artefactual staining of the presynaptic membrane due to diffusion of the enzymatic reaction product of the immunestain cannot be excluded at present.

Labeling of the GABA receptor complex either immunohistochemically or autoradiographically (^{3}H-Ro 15-1788) can be used to identify GABAergic synapses on the light microscopic level (Fig. 2). High densities of receptor were detected in rat brain by both methods e.g. in the cerebral cortex, glomerular and external plexiform layers of the olfactory bulb, islets of Calleja, ventral pallidum, hippocampus, dentate gyrus, superior and inferior colliculi and cerebellum (Richards and Möhler 1984; Schoch et al. 1985). Thus, a high density of GABAergic innervation is present in these structures. Low densities of the GABA receptor complex were found in the corpus callosum, parts of the thalamus, pons and medulla (Fig. 2).

The intensity of benzodiazepine radiolabeling and immunostaining differed only in the granular layer of the cerebellum and in the ventro-lateral thalamus. Whether this is due to a structural or a conformational heterogeneity of the receptor complex in these two regions remains to be clarified.

5. Outlook

1. *Genetics:* New information on the synthesis, assembly and structure of the receptor is expected to emerge from the isolation and analysis of the GABA receptor genes. Such studies will also provide DNA probes to identify, by in situ hybridization, the target cells of GABAergic regulation.
2. *Diagnostics:* Possible dysfunction of the GABA receptor complex in CNS diseases can now be monitored immunohistochemically in post mortem human brain. Furthermore, positron emission tomography using ^{11}C-labeled benzodiazepines may allow the detection of receptor abnormalities in human brain in vivo.
3. *Physiology:* The physiological role of the BZR is yet unknown. The functional relevance of an endogenous peptide interacting with BZR (Alho et al. 1985) remains to be established.

Acknowledgments. We thank Dr. W. Haefely for critical reading of the manuscript.

References

Alho H, Costa E, Ferrero P, Fujimoto M, Cosenza-Murphy D, Guidotti A (1985) Diazepam binding inhibitor (DBI): a neuropeptide located in selected neuronal populations of rat brain. Science 229:179–182

Chang L-R, Barnard EA (1982) The benzodiazepine GABA receptor complex: molecular size in brain synaptic membranes and in solution. J Neurochem 39:1507–1518

Haefely W (1985) Pharmacology of benzodiazepine antagonists. Pharmacopsychiatry 18:163–166

Haefely W, Polc P (1985) Electrophysiological studies on the interactions of anxiolytic drugs with GABAergic mechanisms. In: Olsen RW, Venter JC (eds) Benzodiazepine/GABA receptors and chloride channels: structural and functional properties. Alan R. Liss, New York (in press)

Häring P, Stähli C, Schoch P, Takacs B, Staehelin T, Möhler H (1985) Monoclonal antibodies reveal structural homogeneity of γ-aminobutyric acid/benzodiazepine receptors in different brain areas. Proc Natl Acad Sci USA 82:4837–4841

Möhler H, Okada T (1977) Demonstration of benzodiazepine receptors in the central nervous system. Science 198:849–851

Möhler H, Battersby MK, Richards JG (1980) Benzodiazepine receptor protein identified and visualized in brain tissue by a photoaffinity label. Proc Natl Acad Sci USA 77:1666–1670

Möhler H, Richards JG, Wu JY (1981) Autoradiographical localization of benzodiazepine receptors in immunocytochemically identified γ-aminobutyrergic synapses. Proc Natl Acad Sci USA 78:1935–1938

Möhler H, Schoch P, Richards JG, Häring P, Takacs B, Stähli C (1985) Monoclonal antibodies as probes for studying the structure and location of the GABA receptor/benzodiazepine receptor/chloride channel complex. In: Olsen RW, Venter JC (eds) Benzodiazepine/GABA receptors and chloride channels: structural and functional properties. Alan R. Liss, New York (in press)

Richards JG, Möhler H (1984) Benzodiazepine receptors. Neuropharmacology 23:233–242

Schoch P, Häring P, Takacs B, Stähli C, Möhler H (1984) A GABA/benzodiazepine receptor from bovine brain: purification, reconstitution and immunological characterization. J Recept Res 4: 189–200

Schoch P, Richards JG, Häring P, Takacs B, Stähli C, Staehelin T, Haefely W, Möhler H (1985) Co-localization of $GABA_A$ receptors and benzodiazepine receptors in the brain shown by monoclonal antibodies. Nature 314:168–171

Sigel E, Barnard EA (1983) A γ-aminobutyric acid/benzodiazepine receptor complex of bovine cerebral cortex: purification and partial characterization. J Biol Chem 258:6965–6971

Squires RF, Braestrup C (1977) Benzodiazepine receptors in rat brain. Nature 266:732–734

TBPS Binding to the GABA/Benzodiazepine Receptor Complex in Cultured Cerebellar Granule Cells

V. GALLO[1], B.C. WISE[2], F. VACCARINO[2], and A. GUIDOTTI[2]

t-Butylbicyclophosphorothionate (TBPS) is a byciclophosphate derivative with potent picrotoxin-like convulsant activity that binds with high affinity and specificity to a Cl^- channel modulatory site of the GABA/benzodiazepine receptor complex (Squires and Casida 1983). Using intact and differentiated cerebellar granule cells maintained in culture (Kingsbury et al. 1985), we have studied the modifications induced by GABA and diazepam on the ion channel modulatory binding site labeled by (^{35}S)TBPS. Both autoradiographic (Mohler et al. 1981) and biochemical studies (Allen and Dutton 1984) have previously indicated that cerebellar granule cells possess a high density of GABA and benzodiazepine receptors in vivo or in culture. Granule cell-enriched primary cultures and their crude membrane preparations show both GABA and benzodiazepine high affinity, saturable binding sites (Meier and Schousboe 1982).

(^{35}S)TBPS binding to intact granule cell cultures were saturated at concentrations of TBPS higher than 200 nM and represented approximately 70% of the total binding. Nonspecific binding was taken as (^{35}S)TBPS bound to the cells in the presence of 10^{-4} M unlabeled TBPS or picrotoxin. The K_d value was 100 nM and the B_{max} was 440 fmoles/mg prot. Specific (^{35}S)TBPS binding was blocked by unlabeled TBPS, picrotoxin and n-butylbicyclophosphate. The K_i values for these compounds were 0.094, 0.230 and 6.410 μM, respectively. Neither cerebellar astroglial-enriched cultures, nor the NB-2A neuroblastoma cell line exhibited any specific (^{35}S)TBPS binding (data not shown). The Hill coefficient of TBPS binding to granule cells was 1.18, suggesting the presence of only one class of binding sites. In a subsequent serie of experiment we studied the relationship among GABA, benzodiazepine and TBPS binding sites in intact cultured cerebellar cells. (^{35}S)TBPS binding was increased by muscimol, the maximal effect being observed at muscimol concentrations in the range of 1 to 5 μM (Fig. 1). Moreover, bicuculline caused a dose-dependent inhibition of TBPS binding in the concentration range of 0.1–5 μM (85% of inhibition at 5 μM). Bicuculline changed the receptor density rather than the affinity of TBPS for its recognition sites. K_d and B_{max} values were 95 nM and 420 fmoles/mg prot respectively, in the absence of bicuculline, 98 nM and 270 fmoles/mg prot in the presence of 0.5 μM bicuculline. Muscimol reversed the inhibition produced by bicuculline (Fig. 1),

1 Present address: Laboratory of Physiopathology, Istituto Superiore di Sanità, Rome, Italy
2 National Institute of Mental Health, Laboratory of Preclinical Pharmacology, Saint Elizabeths Hospital, Washington, DC 20032, USA

Molecular Aspects of Neurobiology
(ed. by Rita Levi Montalcini et al.)
© Springer-Verlag Berlin Heidelberg 1986

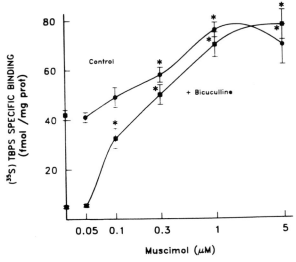

Fig. 1. Muscimol-induced enhancement of (^{35}S)TBPS binding in cultures treated with and without bicuculline. Cerebellar neuronal cultures were prepared and maintained as previously described (Kingsbury et al. 1985). (^{35}S)TBPS binding studies were performed as described elsewhere (Gallo et al. 1985). Bicuculline was 5 μM. Each *point* is the mean ± S.E.M. of 8 dishes from two different cultures. The *asterisks* indicate $p < 0.05$ when compared to respective controls

but failed to reverse the inhibition caused by 5 μM picrotoxin. TBPS binding was also modulated by benzodiazepine receptor ligands. Table 1 shows a 28% stimulation of (^{35}S)TBPS binding induced by 10^{-6} M diazepam and a 34% decrease in binding induced by 10^{-6} M 6,7-dimethoxy-4-ethyl-beta-carboline-3-carboxylic acid methylester (DMCM). The β-carboline RO 15-1788, a postulated benzodiazepine antagonist (Hunkeler et al. 1981), failed to stimulate or to inhibit TBPS binding per se, but antagonized the stimulatory action of diazepam or the inhibitory effect of DMCM (Table 1). In another group of experiments we found that 0.05 μM muscimol failed to reverse bicu-

Table 1. Modulation by benzodiazepine receptor ligands of (^{35}S)TBPS binding to intact cerebellar granule cells

Additions	(^{35}S)TBPS binding (fmol/mg prot)	
	Contr	RO 15-1788 (10 μM)
Control (Solvent)	49 ± 3.0	40 ± 3.5
Diazepam (1 μM)	54 ± 2.2[a]	39 ± 1.5
DMCM (1 μM)	28 ± 1.0[a]	40 ± 3.5

Eight-day-old cultures were incubated with 15 nM (^{35}S)TBPS and the various additions. Each point is the mean ± S.E.M. obtained from a total of eight dishes processed in two separate experiments.

[a] $p < 0.01$ when compared with control

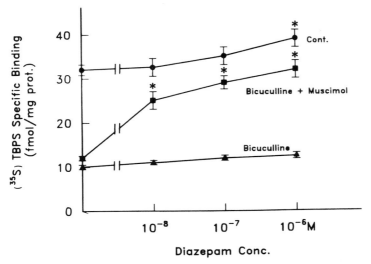

Fig. 2. Potentiation by diazepam of (^{35}S)TBPS binding to cerebellar granule cells in culture. Cells were incubated with solvent (control), 5 μM bicuculline methiodide or 5 μM bicuculline + 0.05 μM muscimol prior to the addition of 10 nM (^{35}S)TBPS. Each value is the mean of nine samples from three different cultures. The *asterisks* indicate $p < 0.05$ when compared with respective controls

culline inhibition of TBPS binding in the absence of diazepam, but it became effective in the presence of 0.1–1 μM diazepam (Fig. 2). These concentrations of diazepam were per se ineffective on TBPS binding (Fig. 2). Also the potentiating effect of diazepam was blocked by RO 15-1788 (Table 2). In cell cultures treated with 5 μM bicuculline, the dose-response curve of muscimol stimulation of TBPS binding was shifted to the left in the presence of 1 μM diazepam; however, the maximum of the curve was not increased (data not shown).

Table 2. Blockade by RO 15-1788 of diazepam plus muscimol-induced increase of (^{35}S)TBPS binding in cerebellar cells incubated with bicuculline

		(^{35}S)TBPS binding (fmol/mg prot)	
Additions	Contr	Bicuculline + Muscimol	Bicuculline + Muscimol + RO 15-1788
Control (Solvent)	48 ± 4.2	19 ± 0.5	17 ± 0.5
Diazepam (0.1 μM)	45 ± 2.0	30 ± 3.5[a]	18 ± 0.8
Diazepam (1 μM)	60 ± 3.8[a]	41 ± 4.5	16 ± 1.0

Eight day old cultures were incubated with 15 nM (^{35}S)TBPS. Each point is the mean ± S.E.M. of six dishes processed in two separate experiments. Bicuculline methiodide (5 μM), muscimol (0.05 μM) and RO 15-1788 (10 μM) were added together with (^{35}S)TBPS.

[a] $p < 0.01$ when compared to the respective groups of controls

These results indicate that the granule cell-enriched cerebellar cultures represent an useful system to study the molecular mechanisms regulating the GABA/benzodiazepine/Cl^- ionophore receptor complex in a homogeneous and intact population of neurons. We have found in the present study that cerebellar granule cells maintained in culture contain a binding site for TBPS, a Cl^- channel modulatory ligand and that this site is affected by the binding of GABA and benzodiazepine to their recognition sites. Our results would suggest that GABA and its agonists unmask and bicuculline masks TBPS binding sites at the cell membrane surface. A possible interpretation of this set of facts is that in the absence of receptor occupancy by GABA the binding sites for TBPS are buried in the cell membrane, perhaps in association with closed channels. TBPS binding sites would become available at the membrane surface when GABA occupies its receptor, the activation of which leads to the opening of the Cl^- channel.

References

Allen AJ, Dutton GR (1984) ^{3}H-Fluinitrazepam binding to neurone-enriched cerebellar cultures. Pharmacologist 26:180

Gallo V, Wise BC, Vaccarino F, Guidotti A (1985) GABA and benzodiazepine-induced modulation of (^{35}S)-t-butylbicyclophosphorothionate binding to cerebellar granule cells. J Neurosci 5: 2432–2438

Hunkeler W, Mohler H, Pieri L, Polc P, Bonetti EP, Cumin R, Schaffner R, Haefely W (1981) Selective antagonists of benzodiazepines. Nature 290:514–516

Kingsbury AE, Gallo V, Woodhams PL, Balazs R (1985) Survival, morphology and adhesion properties of cerebellar interneurones cultured in chemically-defined and serum-supplemented media. Dev Brain Res 17:17–25

Meier E, Schousboe A (1982) Differences between GABA receptor binding to membranes from cerebellum during postnatal development and from cultured cerebellar granule cells. Dev Neurosci 5:546–553

Mohler H, Richards JG, Wu JY (1981) Autoradiographic localization of benzodiazepine receptors in immunocytochemically identified gamma aminobutyrergic synapses. Proc Natl Acad Sci USA 78:1935–1938

Squires RF, Casida JE, Richardson ME, Saederup E (1983) ^{35}S-t-butylbicyclophosphorothionate binds with high affinity to brain specific sites coupled to gamma aminobutyric acid-A and ion recognition sites. Mol Pharmacol 23:326–336

Distribution and Transmembrane Organization of Glycine Receptors at Central Synapses: an Immunocytochemical Touch

A. TRILLER[1], F. CLUZEAUD[1], F. PFEIFFER[2], and H. KORN[1]

1. Introduction

Immunocytochemistry now provides a powerful tool to address questions as (1) the exact localization of central receptors in relation to their corresponding sites of transmitter release and (2) the transmembrane organization of the determinants recognized by monoclonal antibodies (mAbs). It overcomes the lack of specific ligands such as α-bungarotoxine, which permitted the structure of peripheral acetylcholine receptors to be unraveled (ref. in Changeux et al. 1984). The problem of raising and characterizing mAbs against identified antigens, such as those directed against the glycine receptors (ref. in Graham et al. 1985) which were used for this work remains. Glycine is a neurotransmitter ubiquitously distributed in the CNS, where it produces a Cl^--dependent postsynaptic inhibition; the similarity of our results obtained with these mAbs in two different structures of phylogenetically remote species allow us to postulate the generality of our observations.

Data reported here are from rat spinal cord and goldfish Mauthner cell (MC). Three mAbs raised against the denatured glycine receptor (ref. in Graham et al. 1985) were selected; they include the mAb GlyR 2b, 5a and 7a, which react against the 48, 93 kD, and both protomeres, respectively. They were visualized with biotin-avidin-HRP technique, or by labeling with colloidal gold particles (5 nm) adsorbed with protein A, following a treatment with rabbit anti-mouse Ig (RAM). Some sections were impregnated with E-PTA for visualization of the presynaptic grid.

2. The Localization and Extension of the Receptors

These were first studied in lamina VIII and IX of the rat, at least in part, on motorneurons (for details, see Triller et al. 1985). The immunoreactive epitopes were concentrated at the postsynaptic side of the synaptic complex (Fig. 1A,C), suggesting a distribution comparable to that observed at the neuromuscular junction where the

1 INSERM U261, Département de Biologie Moléculaire, Institut Pasteur, 25 rue du Doctor Roux, 75724 Paris Cedex 15, France
2 Max-Planck-Institut für Biochemie, Abt. Oesterhelt, 8033 Martinsried, FRG

Molecular Aspects of Neurobiology
(ed. by Rita Levi Montalcini et al.)
© Springer-Verlag Berlin Heidelberg 1986

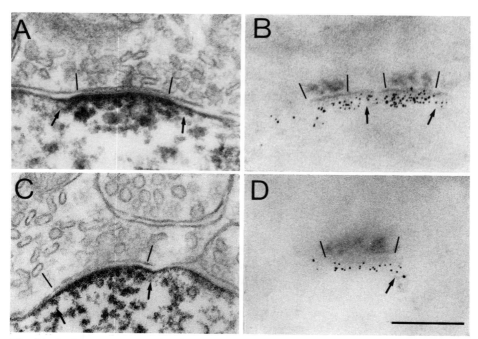

Fig. 1A–D. Immunocytochemical evidence that glycine receptors are localized at synaptic complexes. Transverse views from ventral regions of the rat cervical spinal cord, stained by mAb GlyR 5a (**A, B**) and mAb GlyR 7a (**C, D**). **A, C** The enzymatic reaction product is mostly concentrated at the level of the synaptic complex (delineated by *bars*) identified by the shape of the synaptic cleft. **B, D** Immunogold labeling on semi-thin (0.5 μm) sections impregnated with E-PTA, for staining of the presynaptic active zones (*between bars*); the two in **B** may be an annular one. Note that in all cases the determinants (*arrows*) extend slightly over the limits of the latter. Calibration: 200 nm

highest density of receptors faces the release sites. Their domain (i.e., the "receptor matrix") was better delineated with immunogold labeling associated to E-PTA staining which further showed that they extend slightly beyond the limit of the synaptic complex (Fig. 1B,D).

Recently, these results were extended by observations made at the level of the MC axon cap (Fig. 2A), where inhibitory synapses, which can be identified morphologically (Nakajima 1974; ref. in Faber and Korn 1978), produce a powerful IPSP presumed to be mediated by glycine (Fig. 2B1, B2; see also Faber and Korn 1978). In confirmation, the immunoenzymatic reaction was found in front of the active zones of some small vesicle boutons (Fig. 2C) and of unmyelinated club endings, outside and within the AC (Fig. 2D,E), respectively. Their localization (Fig. 2D), with respect to the active zones, was the same as in rat and, despite a slight overextension of their boundaries, there was no confluence of the domains of adjacent terminals (Fig. 2E). Thus the proposition that the receptor matrix involved in the generation of the MC-IPSP is widely distributed (Faber et al. 1985) is only confirmed in fact by this approach, which may however fail to detect low concentrations of antigens.

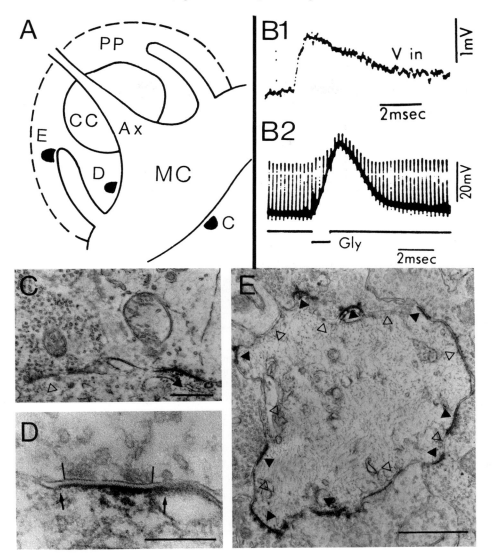

Fig. 2A–E. Visualization of glycine receptors on the Mauthner (MC) cell. **A** Schematic drawing of the axon cap which surrounds the initial segment of the MC axon (*Ax*) showing its limits (*dashed line*), central core (*CC*), and peripheral part (*PP*). **C–E** Indicate the localization of the synapses illustrated in the corresponding plates below. **B1–B2** Electrophysiological presumptions for the glycinergic nature of the M-cell chemical inhibition. **B1** Mean unitary inverted IPSP (n = 8) evoked by impulses in a presynaptic interneuron. **B2** Increased membrane conductance due to iontophoretically applied glycine, shown by the reduction in antidromic spike height. (Modified from Faber and Korn 1982, with permission). **C–E** Immunoenzymatic characterization of receptor areas, with mAb GlyR 5a. Note the discontinuous aspect of the staining indicated by alternation of labeled (*filled triangles*) and unlabeled (*open triangles*) patches of membrane. The higher magnification in **D** suggests that the receptive region is larger than the corresponding presynaptic active zone (same symbols as for Fig. 1). (Calibration bars: 0.5, 0.2, and 1 μm for **C**, **D** and **E**, respectively)

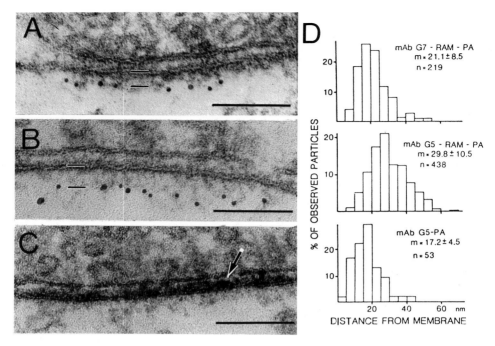

Fig. 3A–D. Transmembrane localization of some antigenic determinants in the rat spinal cord. **A, B** Transverse sections of active zones stained by gold particles indirectly linked to mAb GlyR 7a (**A**) and to mAb GlyR 5a (**B**), showing that the determinants are at the intracellular side of the membrane, and illustrating the distance between them (*small bars*). **C** Evidence that the antigenic determinant recognized by mAb GlyR 2b (immunoenzymatic reaction) is on the extracytoplasmic side of the plasmalemma (*arrow*). (Calibration bars: 100 μm). **D** Frequency histograms of the distance between the membrane and gold particles associated with the indicated mAbs, with (*upper* and *middle*) and without (*lower*) RAM. The mean values between the upper and the lower two histograms (also shown) where statistically different (student t test p < 1‰). Note the reduction in distance when the RAM was not used

3. The Localization of the Determinants with Respect to the Membrane

This can be approached (see Triller et al. 1985) by measurements of the distances between lipidic portion of the membrane and the gold particles, which were not the same for mAb GlyR 7a (Fig. 3A,D, upper histogram) and mAb GlyR 5a (Fig. 3B,D, middle histogram). The results of these computations indicate that although these two determinants are both intracytoplasmic, they have different locations and relationships with the plasmalemma. Furthermore, the size of IGgs used (RAM and mAb) was assessed from labeling in absence of RAM (Fig. 3D, lower part). By subtraction, one could estimate the protrusion in the cytoplasm of the epitope recognized by GlyR 5a to be about 5–8 nm, which is similar to the extracellular protrusion of the acetylcholine receptor (ref. in Changeux 1984). On the other hand, mAb GlyR 2b directed against the

48 kD subunit, which bears the glycine binding site, recognizes an extracellular membranous determinant (Fig. 3C).

Acknowledgments. We thank Dr. C. Sotelo (INSERM U106, Foch, Suresnes) for providing EM facilities and A. Ryter (Institut Pasteur, Paris) for colloidal gold-protein A. We are indebted to H. Betz (ZMBH, Heidelberg) for providing us with monoclonal antibodies against glycine receptors. This work was supported by grants from INSERM (Paris, France) and Deutsche Forschungsgemeinschaft (Grant no. BE 718/6-6).

References

Changeux JP, Devillers-Thiéry A, Chemouilli P (1984) Acetylcholine receptor: an allosteric protein. Science 225:1335–1345

Faber DS, Korn H (1978) Electrophysiology of the Mauthner cell: basic properties, synaptic mechanisms and associated network. In: Faber DS, Korn H (eds) Neurobiology of the Mauthner cell, 47–131

Faber DS, Korn H (1982) Transmission at a central inhibitory synapse. I – Magnitude of unitary postsynaptic conductance change and kinetics of channel activation. J Neurophysiology 48: 654–678

Faber DS, Funch PG, Korn H (1985) Evidence that receptors mediating central synaptic potential extend beyond the postsynaptic density. Proc Natl Acad Sci USA 82:3504–3508

Graham D, Pfeiffer F, Simler R, Betz H (1985) Purification and characterization of the glycine receptor of pig spinal cord. Biochemistry 24:990–994

Triller A, Cluzeaud F, Pfeiffer F, Betz H, Korn H (1985) Distribution of glycine receptors at central synapses: an immuno-electron microscopy study. J Cell Biol 101:683–688

Modulation of a Potassium Channel in *Aplysia* Sensory Neurons: Role of Protein Phosphorylation

J.S. CAMARDO, M.J. SHUSTER, and S.A. SIEGELBAUM[1]

1. Introduction

Serotonin (5-HT) produces a slow depolarizing postsynaptic potential in the mechano-receptor sensory neurons of the abdominal ganglia of the marine snail *Aplysia*. This slow EPSP is accompanied by a decrease in resting membrane conductance, a broadening of the action potential duration, and an increase in transmitter release from the sensory neuron terminals. The increase in transmitter release is thought to underlie behavioral sensitization of the gill-withdrawal reflex (Kandel and Schwartz 1982). Voltage clamp experiments have shown that the primary effect of serotonin in the sensory neurons is to decrease a specific outward potassium membrane current (S current) that is distinct from the previously identified K^+ currents in molluscan neurons (Klein et al. 1982).

There is now good evidence that the modulatory effects of serotonin on the S current are mediated by the second messenger cyclic AMP acting via cAMP-dependent protein phosphorylation (Kandel and Schwartz 1982), according to the following general scheme (Krebs 1972): 1. The binding of 5-HT to its receptor leads to activation of membrane bound adenylate cyclase. 2. This leads to a rise in intracellular cAMP. 3. cAMP than activates cAMP-dependent protein kinase (cAMP-PK). 4. The catalytic subunit of protein kinase phosphorylates several substrate proteins. 5. This leads to the decrease in S current by some unknown mechanism.

While a good deal is known about the mechanism of conventional transmitter actions at the molecular level of single ion channel function (e.g., the action of acetyl-choline at the nicotinic receptor; Colquhoun and Sakmann 1983), much less is known about how modulatory cAMP-dependent transmitter actions alter ion channel behavior. Towards this end, we have used single channel recording (Hamill et al. 1981) to investigate the mechanism of action of serotonin in *Aplysia* sensory neurons. Our interests were first to identify the serotonin-sensitive potassium channel, then to characterize the mode of action of 5-HT on single channel function, and finally to investigate the link between protein phosphorylation and channel modulation using cell-free membrane patches.

1 Departments of Pharmacology and Physiology, Center for Neurobiology and Behavior, College of Physicians and Surgeons, Columbia University, 722 West 168th Street, New York, NY 10032, USA

Molecular Aspects of Neurobiology
(ed. by Rita Levi Montalcini et al.)
© Springer-Verlag Berlin Heidelberg 1986

From the previous voltage clamp studies on serotonin's action in the sensory neurons, it was clear that the net effect of serotonin was to reduce the total outward S potassium current (Klein et al. 1982). At the level of single channel function, this overall effect could be produced in several ways. The total average macroscopic S current, I_S, is given by: $I_S = N_f*p*i$, where N_f is the number of functional S channels in the membrane, p in the probability that a given channel is open, and i is the amplitude of the current flow through a single open S channel. Serotonin could then cause a reduction in I_S by reducing the single channel conductance so that less current flows through an open channel (decreased i), by reducing the probability that a channel is open (decreased p), or by preventing a certain fraction of channels from opening, which would appear as a decrease in the number of functional channels in the membrane (decreased N_f).

2. Serotonin Closes a Specific Potassium Channel

To investigate the mode of serotonin's action on single S channels, we obtained single channel current recordings from sensory neurons using a fire-polished patch pipette that was tightly sealed against the sensory cell surface. Figure 1 illustrates the action of serotonin on single S channel currents from a patch that initially contained four active S channels. Figure 1A shows the action of serotonin on a slow time scale. Figure 1B shows the current record before application of serotonin using a faster time scale which allows us to resolve the rapid opening and closing of these channels. At a membrane potential of 0 mV, channel openings contribute square outward going pulses of current with an amplitude of around 4 pA. The current record jumps up and down among a number of descrete levels due to the random openings and closings of the four channels. Since the amplitudes of the unit current steps are relatively uniform from one channel opening to the next, we can reasonably conclude that the four channels represent a single population of channels.

Figure 1A shows the onset of 5-HT action on channel currents on a slower time scale. At the arrow, 100 μM 5-HT was added to the bath. Within a few seconds after addition of transmitter, there was a small depolarization in the sensory neuron resting potential and a decrease in resting conductance (data not shown). At the same time, the single channel current record shows a slow stepwise decrease in channel activity as three of the four active channels close in an all-or-none manner in response to 5-HT. Figure 1C shows a record of single channel current on a faster time scale which illustrates that, in the presence of 5-HT, the remaining active channel appears to function normally, with an unaltered single channel conductance and probability of opening. Thus, serotonin does not promote the appearance of channel currents with reduced conductance or with an altered probability of opening. Rather, serotonin appears to cause long-lasting channel closures which results in an apparent decrease in the number of functional channels in the membrane.

This result also provides indirect support that the effects of serotonin are mediated by an intracellular messenger. In these experiments, 5-HT is applied to the cell only after formation of the high resistance seal. This tight contact between the glass pipette

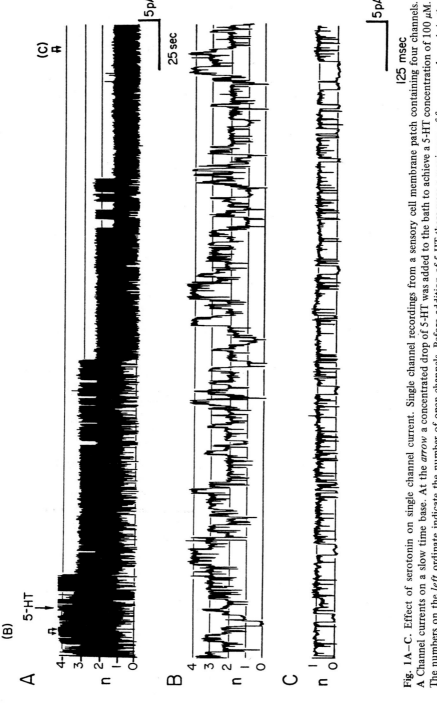

Fig. 1A–C. Effect of serotonin on single channel current. Single channel recordings from a sensory cell membrane patch containing four channels. **A** Channel currents on a slow time base. At the *arrow* a concentrated drop of 5-HT was added to the bath to achieve a 5-HT concentration of 100 μM. The numbers on the *left* ordinate indicate the number of open channels. Before addition of 5-HT there were a maximum of four open channels in the patch. The *small arrows* labeled (**B**) and (**C**) indicate regions of trace A from which expanded records shown in traces **B** and **C** were obtained. Cell resting potential was −41 mV before 5-HT. In presence of 5-HT the cell depolarized to −37 mV and there was a 33% increase in membrane resistance. Patch membrane potential = 0 mV before 5-HT and +4 mV after 5-HT

and the cell membrane prevents the diffusion of 5-HT from the bath into the pipette, thus making it likely that some intracellular messenger mediates the action of 5-HT. Direct support for this scheme has been obtained in experiments where injection of cAMP into sensory neurons from cAMP-filled microelectrodes has been shown to mimic the effects of serotonin in closing the channels.

In other experiments we have further characterized the single channel properties of the S channel. We find that the channel is at least 10-fold selective for potassium ions over sodium ions. Channel opening is independent of intracellular calcium and only moderately sensitive to changes in membrane potential. Since the channel is open at both the resting potential and at more depolarized potentials, it will contribute outward hyperpolarizing current to help set the level of the normal resting potential and aid in repolarization of the action potential. Closure of such a channel can thus explain the slow decreased conductance EPSP as well as spike broadening produced by serotonin in the sensory neurons.

3. cAMP-Dependent Protein Kinase Closes the S Channel in Cell-Free Patches

One major question concerning all cAMP-dependent transmitter actions, including closure of the S channel, is the nature of the link between protein phosphorylation and channel modulation. While the most direct mechanism for S channel closure involves phosphorylation of the channel by protein kinase, there are several plausible alternatives involving phosphorylation of various membrane bound or cytoplasmic intermediary proteins. At present, despite the wide variety of transmitter actions that are known to be mediated by cAMP-dependent protein phosphorylation (see Nestler and Greengard 1983), very little is known about the identity or subcellular localization of any of the substrate phosphoproteins that control channel activity. Moreover, while several groups have demonstrated an effect of the catalytic subunit of protein kinase on cellular electrophysiological properties (Nestler and Greengard 1983), there has been no characterization of the effects of kinase on single channel currents.

We have studied the action of cAMP-PK on S channels in cell-free patches of membrane to determine whether kinase can modulate the channels under such simplified in vitro conditions. Single channel currents were recorded from cell-free inside-out patches of membrane (where the cytoplasmic surface of the membrane faces the bath solution) by withdrawing the patch pipette from the cell surface after formation of the high resistance seal. Our results show that the purified catalytic subunit of cAMP-PK in the presence of MgATP causes prolonged all-or-none channel closures. Figure 2 shows the results of one experiment where kinase was applied to an inside-out patch where there were initially four channels active (Fig. 2A). After addition of the catalytic subunit, a maximum of two of the four active channels closed (Fig. 2B). The channels that remain active appear unchanged with a normal single channel current amplitude and normal open probability. Upon washing the kinase out of the bath, channel activity returned to its initial level (Fig. 2C).

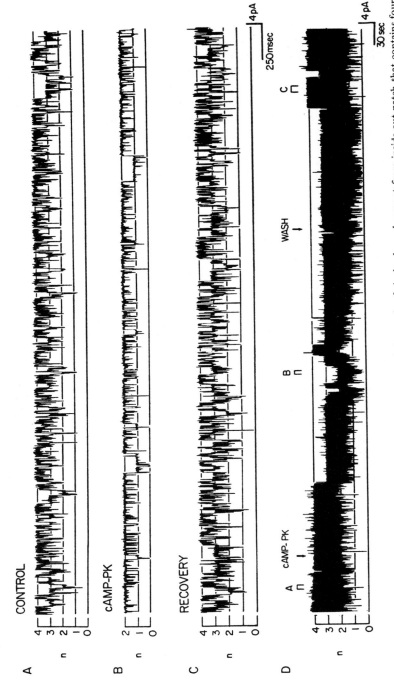

Fig. 2A–D. Effect of cAMP-PK on S channel currents. **A–C** Expanded records of single channel current from inside-out patch that contains four active S channels. **A** Before addition of kinase four S channels are active and open for most of the time. **B** Three minutes after addition of 0.1 μM of the purified catalytic subunit of cAMP-dependent protein kinase (in the presence of 2 mM MgATP) two of the four channels have closed. However, the remaining two channels have a normal single channel amplitude and open probability. **C** After washing kinase out of the bath channel activity recovers to its initial level. **D** Effects of cAMP-PK on channel activity shown on a slower time scale. *Arrows* indicate time of addition of cAMP-PK to the bath and time of washout. Expanded records in A–C taken from times indicated by *brackets*. Membrane potential was held at 0 mV in this experiment

These prolonged all-or-none S channel closures produced by kinase in cell-free patches resemble the closures produced by 5-HT in cell-attached patches. The closures are mediated by a phosphorylation reaction since in the absence of MgATP, the source of high energy phosphate, kinase is four times less effective in producing channel closures than it is in the presence of MgATP. However, the effects of kinase are not identical to those of 5-HT. Thus, the average fraction of active channels in the patches that are closed by kinase (0.34) is somewhat less than the average fraction of channels closed by 5-HT (0.46). Moreover, the average duration of the kinase-induced closures is shorter than the serotonin-induced closures. With serotonin, the channel closures tend to outlast the period of 5-HT application by several minutes. However with kinase, channels close for an average of 2—3 min and then spontaneously reopen, even in the maintained presence of kinase (Fig. 2D).

These differences could be due to the lack of some component in the cell-free patches that is necessary for full modulation. Alternatively, the weaker action of kinase could be due to the presence of active phosphoprotein phosphatase in the cell-free patches. Some indirect evidence in support of a role for phosphatase comes from our finding that fluoride ions, a non-specific phosphatase inhibitor, consistently potentiate the effects of kinase. Fluoride (20—50 mM) increases the fraction of channels closed by kinase from 0.34 to 0.49 and also prolongs the mean duration of channel closure several fold.

The finding that the purified catalytic subunit of cyclic AMP-dependent protein kinase produces all-or-none channel closures in cell-free patches further strengthens a role for this enzyme in mediating the action of 5-HT. In addition, it strongly suggests that the critical substrate phosphoprotein that is required for channel modulation is a membrane-associated protein present in the cell-free patches. At this point, however, we cannot determine whether it is the channel itself that is phosphorylated or whether some other protein mediates the action of the kinase. Our results also suggest that the cell-free patches may lack some component necessary for producing long-lasting closures. One possibility is that the membrane patches contain a phosphoprotein phosphatase that is normally inhibited in the intact cell by specific cytoplasmic phosphatase inhibitor proteins (Ingebritsen and Cohen 1983; Hemmings et al. 1984). Experiments testing the effects of these specific inhibitors on the action of kinase in cell-free patches will be useful in future experiments exploring the role of phosphatase in regulating S channel modulation.

References

Colquhoun D, Sakmann B (1983) Bursts of openings in transmitter activated ion channels. In: Sakmann B, Neher E (eds) Single channel recording. Plenum, New York

Hamill OP, Marty A, Neher E, Sakmann B, Sigworth F (1981) Improved patch-clamp techniques for high-resolution current recording from cells and cell-free membrane patches. Pflügers Arch 391:85—100

Hemmings HC, Greengard P, Lim Tung HY, Cohen P (1984) DARPP-32$_1$, a dopamine-regulated neuronal phosphoprotein, is a potent inhibitor of protein phosphatase-1. Nature 310:503—505

Ingebritsen TS, Cohen P (1983) Protein phosphatases: properties and role in cellular regulation. Science 221:331−337

Kandel ER, Schwartz JH (1982) Molecular biology of learning: Modulation of transmitter release. Science 218:433−443

Klein M, Camardo JS, Kandel ER (1982) Serotonin modulates a specific potassium current in the sensory neurons that show presynaptic facilitation in *Aplysia*. Proc Natl Acad Sci USA 79: 5713−5717

Krebs EG (1972) Protein kinases. Curr Top Cell Regul 5:99−133

Nestler EJ, Greengard P (1983) Protein phosphorylation in the brain. Nature 305:583−588

Siegelbaum SA, Camardo JS, Kandel ER (1982) Serotonin and cAMP close single K channels in *Aplysia* sensory neurons. Nature 299:413−417

Voltage-gated Sodium, Potassium and Chloride Channels in Rat Cultured Astrocytes

J.M. RITCHIE, S. BEVAN, S.Y. CHIU, and P.T.A. GRAY[1]

Axon-free rabbit degenerating nerve trunks (Ritchie and Rang 1983) avidly bind labeled saxitoxin. Since the main cell population is composed of Schwann cells, which have proliferated to fill the space vacated by the axons, this binding must have been to these PNS satellite cells. Subsequent electrophysiological experiments (Chiu et al. 1984; Shrager et al. 1985) have shown that Schwann cells indeed express plasmalemmal voltage-sensitive sodium channels. We now show that CNS satellite cells, the astrocytes, also bind saxitoxin and express plasmalemmal voltage-dependent sodium channels. Furthermore, like the PNS Schwann cells they also express voltage-dependent potassium channels.

Astrocytes were prepared by the method of McCarthy and de Vellis (1980; see also Bevan et al. 1985). Staining with antibodies to GFAP, a known marker for astrocytes, showed that 90% of the cells were GFAP-positive, the remainder being fibroblast-like. Proliferation of these contaminating cells was inhibited by cytosine arabinoside. Single channel and whole-cell currents were recorded with the patch clamp technique from cells usually "rounded" by a 5-min exposure to 0.5 mg/ml trypsin and 0.6 mM EDTA.

Because of the large size of the astrocytes, and because of their irregular shape even after "rounding", clamping conditions were not optimal. Nevertheless, voltage-clamp depolarization of these cells (Fig. 1) clearly produces voltage-dependent inward and

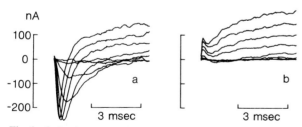

Fig. 1a, b. Ionic currents (leak subtracted) in whole-cell recordings from rat cultured astrocytes. The cells were held at −70 mV, pulsed for 100 ms to −100 mV to remove sodium channel inactivation, and then taken in 10 mV steps to series of potentials between −70 and 0 mV. (Record a is taken before and b after exposure to tetrodotoxin)

1   Department of Pharmacology, Yale University School of Medicine, New Haven, CT 06510, USA

Molecular Aspects of Neurobiology
(ed. by Rita Levi Montalcini et al.)
© Springer-Verlag Berlin Heidelberg 1986

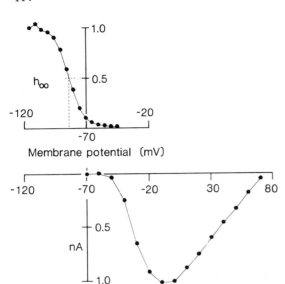

Fig. 2. The h-infinity and peak current-voltage relations for a rat cultured astrocyte

outward currents. Most of the outward current (60–70%) is blocked by TEA, 4-amino-pyridine, or internal caesium and is taken to be a potassium current. The inward current is totally blocked by tetrodotoxin (Fig. 1b) and is taken to be a sodium current. The concentration of toxin required to block the current is relatively high (K_D = 500 nM) compared to that required to produce half-maximal saturation of the saxitoxin binding sites (K_D = 2 nM). It remains a matter of speculation whether or not there is some dynamic equilibrium between these two site populations (the low affinity site determined electrophysiologically and the high affinity site detected by saxitoxin binding).

The peak current-voltage curve and the h-infinity relation of the astrocytic sodium channels are similar to those previously determined for rabbit nodal membrane (Chiu et al. 1979) except that the former is shifted about 30 mV in the depolarizing direction. This shift makes it unlikely that the astrocyte generates an action potential although it has all the machinery for doing so. In the absence of any clear direct function for the astrocyte, we speculate that these voltage-dependent sodium and potassium channels may be synthesized by the astrocyte (where they are inoperative) and subsequently transferred to the axolemma of associated neurons. Such a transfer between the corresponding peripheral satellite cell, the Schwann cell, and the axolemma has already been proposed (Shrager et al. 1985).

On average, only 60–70% of the outward current is blocked by conventional potassium channel blocking agents. The remaining current is a chloride current. Figure 3 (●) shows the peak current-voltage relation at the end of a 100 ms test pulse in a preparation where the classical outward potassium current has already been blocked by caesium chloride in the patch pipette. Replacement of the chloride in the bathing solution by the much larger anion ascorbate (○) immediately blocks this outward current (without affecting the inward sodium current). This effect is rapidly reversed on replacing the ascorbate with chloride. Other anions intermediate in size

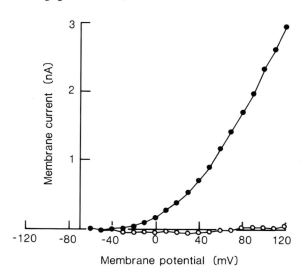

Fig. 3. Peak current-voltage relation from a rat cultured astrocyte (with CsCl in the pipette) in response to depolarizations from a holding potential of −70 mV to +120 mV in 10 mV steps. The bathing medium was either 150 mM NaCl (●) or 150 mM sodium ascorbate (○) and also contained HEPES buffer and 2.2 mM calcium gluconate

between ascorbate and chloride (e.g. isethionate, sulphate) produce intermediate effects.

Since the voltage-dependent chloride conductance is characteristic of the central satellite cell, being small or absent in the Schwann cell, we suggest that it may play a role in the spatial buffering of potassium in the CNS. It has been suggested (for example, see Orkand 1982) that the difference between the potassium equilibrium potentials in a region where the potassium concentration is high (because of neuronal activity) and that in a distant region where the extracellular concentration is lower, drives an uptake of potassium from the region of higher concentration and a release in the region of lower concentration, so permitting more ongoing neuronal activity. By also activating a chloride conductance, the depolarization allows chloride to enter the cell with the potassium, which allows some be stored locally in the glia immediately neighbouring the active neurons rather than being released more remotely. The potassium is thus more readily accessible to the neuron for recapture during recovery. This process, which would be aided by the concomitant voltage-activated increase in the potassium conductance, would supplement rather than replace the previously described distant release. Recent experimental support for this hypothesis comes from the finding that depolarization of invertebrate glial cells by an increase in extracellular potassium concentration does in fact raise the intracellular chloride concentration (Coles et al. 1985).

Acknowledgments. This work was supported in part by grants NS 08304 and NS 12327 from the USPHS, by a grant RD 1162 from the U.S. National Multiple Sclerosis Society, and by travel grants (to S.B. and P.T.A.G.) from the Wellcome Trust.

References

Bevan S, Chiu SY, Gray PTA, Ritchie JM (1985) The presence of voltage-gated sodium, potassium and chloride channels in rat cultured astrocytes. Proc R Soc Lond B 225:299–313

Chiu SY, Ritchie JM, Rogart RB, Stagg D (1979) A quantitative description of membrane currents in rabbit myelinated nerve. J Physiol (Lond) 292:149–161

Chiu SY, Shrager P, Ritchie JM (1984) Neuronal-type Na^+ and K^+ channels in rabbit cultured Schwann cells. Nature (Lond) 311:156–157

Coles JA, Orkand RK, Yamate CL (1985) Chloride enters receptors and glia in response to light or raised external potassium in the retina of the bee drone *Apis mellifera*. Experientia 41:827–828

McCarthy K, de Vellis J (1980) Preparation of separate astroglial and oligodendroglial cell cultures from rat cerebral tissue. J Cell Biol 85:890–902

Orkand RK (1982) Signalling between neuronal and glial cells. In: Sears TA (ed) Neuronal-glial cell interrelationships. Springer, Berlin Heidelberg New York, p 147

Ritchie JM, Rang HP (1983) Extraneuronal saxitoxin binding sites in rabbit myelinated nerve. Proc Natl Acad Sci USA 80:2803–2807

Shrager P, Chiu SY, Ritchie JM (1985) Voltage-dependent sodium and potassium channels in mammalian cultured Schwann cells. Proc Natl Acad Sci USA 82:948–952

Molecular Weights of Subunits of the Na$^+$ Channel and a Ca^{2+}-activated K$^+$ Channel in Rat Brain

M.J. SEAGAR, E. JOVER, and F. COURAUD[1]

1. Introduction

Neurotoxins which specifically modify membrane conductances have been widely used as probes to gain an insight into the structure of ion channels. The voltage sensitive Na$^+$ channel carries four distinct neurotoxin binding sites (Catterall 1984), a property which has facilitated its recent purification and biochemical characterization. In contrast K$^+$ channels, for which almost no high affinity ligands have been discovered, remain practically unexplored at the molecular level.

We have used α and β scorpion toxins (ScTx) which bind to sites 3 and 4, respectively, on the Na$^+$ channel and apamin which binds to a type of Ca^{2+} activated K$^+$ channel to label their receptors in both membranes and primary cultured neurons from the rat brain. The synthesis of photoreactive toxin derivatives has allowed the identification of receptor associated polypeptides and radiation inactivation data has proved complementary by indicating the functional target size of membrane binding sites.

2. Na$^+$ Channel Subunits

Binding studies have shown that ScTx active on the mammalian Na$^+$ channel can be subdivided into two groups (α and β ScTx) each group recognizing a distinct receptor site (sites 3 and 4) with no competitive interaction occuring between the two (Jover et al. 1980). Pharmacological effects are compatible with this observation in that α ScTx prolongs the action potential by slowing down or blocking Na$^+$ channel inactivation whereas β ScTx modifies activation by inducing an abnormal slow inward Na$^+$ current on repolarization (Couraud et al. 1982).

Aryl azide derivatives of a ^{125}I-α ScTx (*Leiurus quinquestriatus quinquestriatus* V) and a ^{125}I-βScTx (*Centruroides suffusus suffusus* VI) bind specifically to sites 3 and 4 on rat brain synaptosomes. Photolysis lead to the specific labeling by both toxins of 270,000 and 35,000 polypeptides (Darbon et al. 1983; Fig. 1a) which probably cor-

1 INSERM U172, CNRS UA 553, Laboratoire de Biochimie, Faculté de Médecine, Secteur Nord, Bd. P. Dramard, 13326 Marseille Cedex 15, France

Molecular Aspects of Neurobiology
(ed. by Rita Levi Montalcini et al.)
© Springer-Verlag Berlin Heidelberg 1986

M.J. Seagar et al.

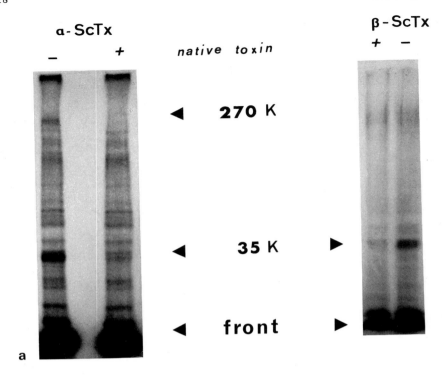

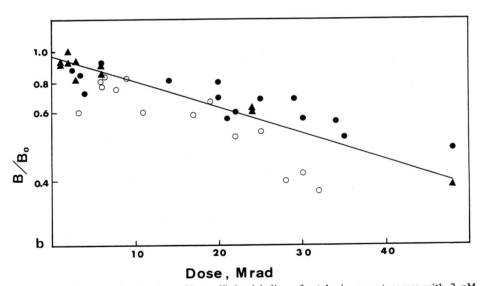

Fig. 1a,b. Na$^+$ channel subunits. **a** Photoaffinity labeling of rat brain synaptosomes with 2 nM ^{125}I-ANPAA-α-ScTx or ^{125}I-ANPAA-β-ScTx. Adjacent lanes show receptor site protection by 2 μM native toxin. **b** Target size analysis of the β-ScTx (^{125}I-Css VI) binding unit. Rat brain synaptosomes were frozen and irradiated with 10 MeV electrons at about $-100°$C. The D_{37} was 52.5 Mrad giving a Mr = 34000

respond to the α and β_1 subunits described in the purified rat brain saxitoxin receptor (Catterall 1984). The distribution of radioactivity between the two subunits was not equivalent, α-ScTx incorporates about 15% into the 270,000 chain and 85% into the 35,000 polypeptide, β-ScTx labels the 270,000 only in a residual manner. The presence of several protease inhibitors did not modify the labeling distribution.

Radiation inactivation data using frozen rat brain membrane samples gives a functional size of 34,000 for the β-ScTx binding unit (Fig. 1b) in reasonable agreement with published results (Angelides et al. 1985) and our photoaffinity experiments. These results indicate that the β-ScTx binding domain is entirely contained within the β_1 Na⁺ channel subunit. The fact that the β_1 subunit is also the major photoaffinity-labeled component on cultued neurons, a system which should be relatively free from proteolytic artefacts upholds this idea and strongly supports the existence of functionally important low molecular weight subunits in the mammalian Na⁺ channel (Jover et al., in prep.).

3. Apamin Sensitive K⁺ Channel Subunits

Apamin, a 2000 dalton neurotoxic peptide from bee venom is a unique high affinity blocker of a type of K⁺ channel. Clues as to its precise pharmacological target were first obtained in peripheral systems. In guinea pig hepatocytes apamin inhibits the K⁺ efflux resulting from Ca²⁺ mobilization induced by α_1 adrenergic agonists and A23187 a Ca²⁺ ionophore (Jenkinson 1981). Electrophysiological work in excitable cells has suggested that apamins central neurotoxicity results from a similar mode of action. In the mouse neuroblastoma NIE-115 nM concentrations specifically block the Ca²⁺ activated slow K⁺ current which underlies the afterhyperpolarization, a current thought to control the frequency of repetitive firing (Hugues et al. 1982).

[125]I-apamin binds to a single class of high affinity sites (KD = $\sim$50 pM, Bmax = 10–20 fmol/mg protein) on both primary cultured neurons and synaptic membranes from the rat brain, and receptor occupancy in neurons has been correlated to partial inhibition of Ca²⁺ activated [86]Rb⁺ efflux (Seagar et al. 1984). [125]I-apamin binding depends on the presence of K⁺ ($K_{0.5}$ $\sim$2 mM) suggesting that the receptor is associated with a physiologically relevant cationic site (Seagar et al. 1984).

Apamin contains two primary amines (α-Cys$_1$ and ϵ-Lys$_4$) neither of which are necessary for biological activity. We have therefore randomly coupled ^{125}I-apamin with a photoreactive aryl azide using an amine directed succinimidyl ester. Photo-reactive ^{125}I-apamin specifically incorporated into major polypeptides of 86,000, 33,000, and 22,000 on cultured neurons and 86,000 and 59,000 on synaptic membranes. The presence of protease inhibitors did not modify the labeling pattern (Seagar et al. 1985; Fig. 2).

Recent work using chemically defined photoprobes indicates that different receptor associated polypeptides are labeled according to the position of the aryl azide group on the apamin molecule, suggesting that the receptor may be situated at the limit between two or more K⁺ channel subunits, although target size analysis suggests that the 86,000 subunit alone carries the apamin binding site (Seagar et al., in press).

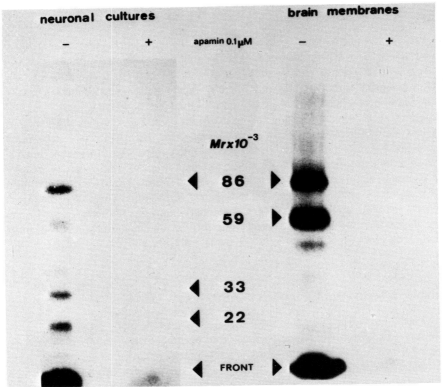

Fig. 2. Apamin-sensitive K⁺ channel subunits. Photoaffinity labeling of neuronal cultures and synaptic membranes from rat brain with 80 pM ¹²⁵I-ANPAA-apamin. Adjacent lanes show receptor site protection by 0.1 μM native apamin

References

Angelides KJ, Nutter TJ, Elmer LW, Kempner ES (1985) Functional unit size of the neurotoxin receptors on the voltage dependent Na⁺ channel. J Biol Chem 260:3431–3439

Catterall WA (1984) The molecular basis of neuronal excitability. Science 223:653–661

Couraud F, Jover E, Dubois JM, Rochat H (1982) Two types of scorpion toxin receptor sites, one related to the activation, the other to the inactivation of the action potential sodium channel. Toxicon 20:9–16

Darbon H, Jover E, Couraud F, Rochat H (1983) Photoaffinity labeling of α- and β-scorpion toxin receptors associated with the rat brain sodium channel. Biochem Biophys Res Commun 115: 415–422

Hugues M, Romey G, Duval D, Vincent JP, Lazdunski M (1982) Apamin as a selective blocker of the calcium dependent potassium channel in neuroblastoma cells: voltage-clamp and biochemical characterization of the toxin receptor. Proc Natl Acad Sci USA 79:1308–1312

Jenkinson DH (1981) Peripheral actions of apamin. Trends Pharmacol Sci 2:318–320

Jover E, Couraud F, Rochat H (1980) Two types of scorpion neurotoxins characterized by their binding to two separate receptor sites on rat brain synaptosomes. Biochem Biophys Res Commun 95:1607–1614

Seagar MJ, Granier C, Couraud F (1984) Interactions of the neurotoxin apamin with a Ca⁺⁺ activated K⁺ channel in primary neuronal cultures. J Biol Chem 259:1491–1495

Seagar MJ, Labbé-Jullié C, Granier C, Van Rietschoten J, Couraud F (1985) Photoaffinity labeling of components of the apamin sensitive K⁺ channel in neuronal membranes. J Biol Chem 260: 3895–3898

Seagar MJ, Labbé-Jullié C, Granier C, Goll A, Glossmann H, Van Rietschoten J, Couraud F (in press) Molecular structure of the rat brain apamin receptor: differential photoaffinity labeling of putative K⁺ channel subunits and target size analysis. Biochemistry

The Differentiation of Cell Types in the Vertebrate CNS

S. HOCKFIELD[1], K. FREDERIKSEN[2], and R. McKAY[2]

1. Introduction

The mechanisms which generate differences between cell types have been a major problem in biology. Every tissue in a eukaryote is made up of a mixture of cell types. The intrinsic molecular properties of these cell types and the interaction between cells gives rise to the specialized functions played by each tissue in an organism. A wide range of newly developed methods are now employed to study the biochemistry of cellular differentiation in eukaryotes.

In neurobiology three new techniques have played a particularly important role in showing that the biochemical diversity of cell types in the nervous system is unexpectedly large. These methods are measurements of message RNA sequence complexity ($C_r$ot analysis), hybridoma and recombinant DNA technology (Cold Spring Harbor Symp 1983). All three techniques lead to the conclusion that a very large number of molecularly distinct cell types cooperate to form the nervous system.

Molecular differences among cells in the nervous system suggest such differences might reflect specialized functions in the nervous system. In the leech we have generated monoclonal antibodies which identify a subset of neurons, those that respond to noxious stimulation of the skin (Zipser and McKay 1981; Johansen et al. 1984). In principle then, molecular markers may be found which identify neurons of a particular functional type. The identification of a functional class of cells by an antibody may be independent of the particular function of the antigen recognized by the antibody. Although an antigen may be related to specific electrophysiological properties of a cell, any single antigenic trait need not be tied to a specific physiological property.

The antibodies used to identify neurons that respond to noxious stimuli in the leech also recognize a subset of axons (Hockfield and McKay 1983a; McKay et al. 1983). These axons travel together in fascicles from the earliest stages of neurite outgrowth. Even at these early stages the axon and its growth cone and filopodia are recognized by the monoclonal antibody (Hockfield and McKay 1983a; McKay et al. 1983). The antigen recognized by the antibody is found on the surface of living cells. Such surface

1 Cold Spring Harbor Laboratory, P.O. Box 100, Cold Spring Harbor, NY 11724, USA
2 Whitaker College and Department of Biology, E25-435, Massachusetts Institute of Technology, Cambridge, MA 02139, USA

Molecular Aspects of Neurobiology
(ed. by Rita Levi Montalcini et al.)
© Springer-Verlag Berlin Heidelberg 1986

chemical differences have been suggested as the basis of the specificity of axon navigation. A number of experiments show that the surface antigens recognized by the antibody are a family of glycoproteins (Hockfield and McKay 1983a; McKay et al. 1983).
The next problem in this series of experiments is to provide direct evidence that these
surface glycoproteins are themselves involved in axon guidance.

This example from the leech illustrates that a specific monoclonal antibody can be
used to analyze both the *cellular* organization of the nervous system and the *biochemical* properties of the specific antigens recognized by that antibody.

The vertebrate nervous system is derived from a group of ectodermal cells which is
induced by the underlying mesoderm to differentiate into the neural plate (Spemann
1938). It is known from transplantation experiments that shortly after mesodermal
induction the ultimate fates of these precursor cells become determined (Chung and
Cooke 1978; Alvarado-Mallart and Sotelo 1984). One feature of this induction is that
the neural plate forms the neural tube. In the neural tube the neuroepithelial cells
proliferate and differentiate to generate arrays of functionally distinct neurons in a
precisely timed sequence (Sidman et al. 1959; Sidman 1970). The neurons migrate
from the proliferative ventricular zone of the neural tube to their adult position where
they extend neurites which navigate to their synaptic targets where synapses are
formed. A number of experiments have shown that the major features of early neural
development take place in the presence of agents which block action potentials (Harris
1980) and are therefore mediated by experience independent process. In contrast, late
events in synaptogenesis are influenced by behavioural experience mediated by action
potentials (Hubel and Wiesel 1970; Hubel et al. 1977; Wiesel and Hubel 1963a,b,
1965, 1985) and represent experience dependent processes.

In this paper we review some of our work in the mammalian CNS where we have
used monoclonal antibodies to explore the molecular basis of the differentiation of
cell types.

2. The Differentiation of Cell Types in Early Neural Tube

On embryonic day 15 (E15) the rat neural tube contains both rapidly proliferating
neural stem cells, radial glial cells, postmitotic neurons migrating away from the
germinal zone and neurons extending axons. In order to obtain markers for the different cell types present at this stage of development, we have generated monoclonal
antibodies directed against cell type specific antigens in the early neural tube (Hockfield and McKay 1985). Mice were immunized with paraformaldehyde-fixed E15
neural tube and monoclonal antibodies were raised by the polyethylene glycol fusion
procedure (Galfre et al. 1977). These antibodies were screeened for those which specifically identified different cell types present in the early neural tube by immunohistochemistry using peroxidase conjugated second antibody on vibratome sections
of paraformaldehyde-fixed E15 neural tube. Two markers for major cell types in the
E15 brain are shown in Fig. 1.

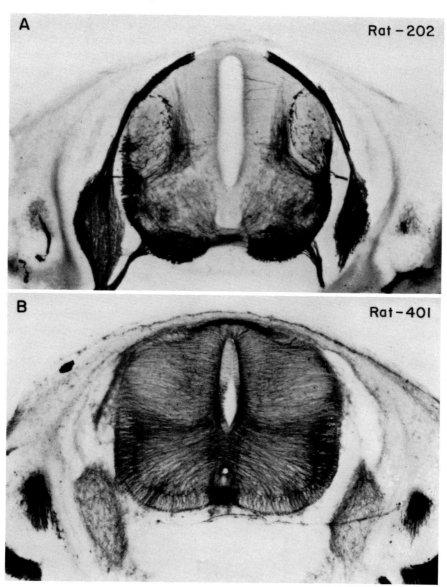

Fig. 1A,B. Immunohistochemistry on sections of the E15 neural tube. Transverse vibratome sections of 4% paraformaldehyde-fixed E15 rat embryos were incubated with mouse monoclonal antibodies (**A** Rat 202; **B** Rat 401). The binding sites of the monoclonal antibodies were visualized with peroxidase conjugated antimouse IgG. Rat 202 binds to axons in the CNS and in the PNS. Rat 401 binds to radial glial cells in the CNS to glial cells in the PNS and to the developing muscle masses

Figure 1A shows the staining pattern of antibody Rat 202 which recognizes axons in the E15 neural tube. The intense staining in the peripheral regions of transverse sections of the neural tube shows the axon rich zone which will become the white matter of the adult spinal cord. Axons can also be seen in the region which contains the cell bodies of post-mitotic motor neurons and in the developing dorsal horn. Many fewer axons are found in the germinal zone immediately adjacent to the ventricle. Rat 202 also recognizes axons in the dorsal and ventral roots of the spinal cord and in the dorsal root ganglia. The staining patterns at the light and electron microscopic levels suggest that all axons are recognized by Rat 202. Silver staining methods and electron microscopy have shown that the first axons appear at E12 in the rat (Windle and Baxter 1936). The timing of Rat 202 expression suggests that this antibody recognizes the first axons. Immunoelectron microscopy shows that Rat 202 recognizes a cytoplasmic antigen in the axons, growth cones and filopodia. On immunoblots Rat 202 recognizes an antigen of 180 kd.

Figure 1B illustrates the staining pattern obtained with the monoclonal antibody Rat 401. In contrast to Rat 202, Rat 401 recognizes cells which extend from the ventricle to the outer pial surface of the neural tube. These cells have the elongated morphology and specialized end feet characteristic of radial glial cells (Cajal Ramon 1972). The appearance of Rat 401 positive cells in the neural tube first occurs after the neural tube has formed while the cells retain their early columnar morphology. Elsewhere in the E15 embryo Rat 401 binds to cells in the peripheral nervous system and in developing muscle masses. Immunoelectron microscopy shows that the antigen is cytoplasmic and is expressed in glial cells in the peripheral nervous system and in developing myotubes. On immunoblots of proteins extracted from the E15 neural tube the antibody binds to a 200 kd band. Rat 401 does not stain any cell type in the adult CNS.

The loss of Rat 401 staining is coincident with the end of the period of neuronal migration. We have shown this correlation between the loss of Rat 401 and the end of the period of neuronal proliferation in the spinal cord and the cerebellum. The molecular weight and the distribution of stained cells in the adult CNS distinguishes the antigen recognized by Rat 401 from glial fibrillary acidic protein (GFAP) and vimentin two other markers of radial glial cells (Dahl et al. 1981; Levitt and Rakic 1980; Levitt et al. 1981; Tapscott et al. 1981).

By late E11 the antigen recognized by Rat 401 is found along the entire ventricular pial extent of the neuro-epithelial cells. Electron-microscopic immunohistochemistry has shown that the Rat-401 antigen does not uniformly fill the neuroepithelial cells at any time. This made it impossible to determine whether all the neuroepithelial cells are Rat 401 positive with in situ immunohistochemical methods. In order to address this question quantitatively we (Frederiksen and McKay, unpubl. data) have developed methods which allow the entire neural tube to be dissected from the rat embryo free of other cell types. The neural tube was dissociated into a single cell suspension with greater than 80% live cells as judged by Trypan blue exclusion and positive staining of live cells with fluorescein diacetate. Small aliquots of these cells were spun down onto coverslips. The total number of cells in the neural tube was calculated by counting the number of nuclei in each aliquot using the fluorescent DNA stain Hoechst 33258. The number of cells of different types was then determined by immunohistochemistry. At

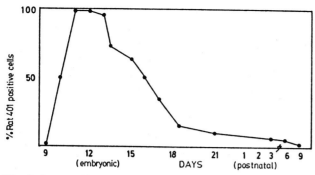

Fig. 2. Immunohistochemistry on dissociated CNS cells through development. Neural tubes were dissected free of other tissue and the cells dissociated. After centrifugation onto a coverslip, the cells were stained with the monoclonal antibody Rat 401 (as in Fig. 1). The percentage of Rat 401 positive cells as a proportion of the total number of cells was seen to increase sharply after E9 to maximum of 98% on E11 and E12 and then decline

E11 to E12 greater than 98% of the cells are Rat 401 positive (Fig. 2). At later times only a subset of cells are Rat 401 positive and 2% are Rat 202 positive. This result suggests that neurons which first appear at E12 are derived from a precursor cell which expresses the Rat 401 antigen.

We have also analyzed cell suspensions stained with specific antibodies by fluorescence activated cell sorting methods. The FACS technique confirms the results obtained by counting stained cells in a fluorescence microscope. In addition the FACS allows quantitative measurement of the DNA content of cells using the fluorescent DNA intercalating dye propidium iodide. Using this method we have shown that a large proportion of Rat 401 positive cells are in the G2 phase of the cell cycle. This result suggests that Rat 401 positive cells are proliferative and confirms immunoelectron-microscopy which shows that Rat 401 positive cells contain mitotic figures.

The fact that the great majority of early neuroepithelial cells express an antigenic marker of radial glial cells suggests that the neuroepithelium first differentiates to generate a population of radial glial cells. Subsequently these radial glial cells generate postmitotic neurons and it is at this time that neuronal markers may be first expressed.

3. The Role of Glial Cells in Axon Elongation

There is considerable evidence that neuronal migration (Rakic 1971, 1976, 1981) and axon elongation (Singer et al. 1979; Silver and Sidman 1980; Nordlander et al. 1981) in the CNS occur on a surface provided by radial glial cells. In contrast to mammals, amphibia can regenerate their CNS and retain radial glial cells in all parts of their CNS into adulthood. In mammals the block to central regeneration can be overcome by providing pathways derived from peripheral nerve (Aguayo et al. 1979). The implication of these studies is that peripheral mammalian nerves retain a glial cell capable of

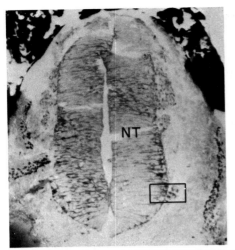

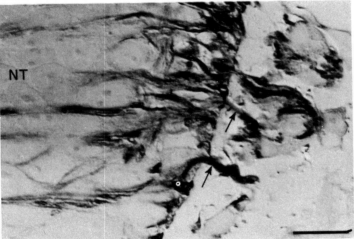

Fig. 3. Immunohistochemistry of Rat 401 on E11 neural tube sections. At this stage of development, before neurons have become postmitotic, Rat 401 positive processes can be seen spanning the boundary between the neural tube and the periphery in the region of the presumptive ventral nerve root (*arrows*)

supporting axon elongation and the CNS loses the glial cell with this function which is present in the embryo.

At E15, Rat 401 recognizes cells in the peripheral nerves and in developing muscle masses. Immuno electron microscopy has shown that in the developing nerve, Rat 401 binds to non-neuronal cells which are likely to be Schwann cell precursors. In the adult peripheral nerve, Rat 401 recognizes Schwann cells and in cultures of peripheral nerve, Rat 401 recognizes Schwann cells and not fibroblasts (Friedman and Hockfield, unpubl. data).

Several observations suggest that the distribution of the Rat 401 antigen in the peripheral nervous system and in the developing central nervous system correlates with glial cells which are capable of supporting axon elongation and neuronal migration. The antigen is expressed in cells in the CNS and PNS during embryonic axon out-growth. Antigen positive cells are lost from the adult CNS but are retained in the PNS. The loss of Rat 401 positive central cells occurs at the end of the period of neuronal migration. This loss of Rat 401 positive cells occurs even in areas of the CNS, such as the cerebellum, which retain radial cells in the adult.

In the early development of the CNS, at E11 in the rat there is a time when the majority of neuroepithelial cells express Rat 401 and neurons have not yet differenti-ated except in the most advanced levels of the neural tube. At this time cross-sections of the neural tube show Rat 401 positive processes which span the CNS boundary in the position of the presumptive ventral nerve roots (Fig. 3).

These results suggest that Rat 401 marks a form of glial cell which can support axon elongation, and that these glial cells in the absence of axons have the ability to detect the pathways which axons will subsequently follow. Another possibility raised by the presence of glial cell processes spanning the pial surface of the neural tube is that some peripheral glial cells are derived from the CNS directly.

4. The Molecular Differentiation of Axons

The antibody Rat 202 is expressed in postmitotic neurons from the earliest stages of neurite outgrowth and throughout adult life. We have raised several antibodies which recognize adult axonal antigens which comigrate with the heavy subunit of the neuro-filament triplet. The antigens recognized by these antibodies are found in neuronal subsets (McKay and Hockfield 1982; Ogren et al. 1985). We have examined the time course of expression of the antigens recognized by these antibodies.

Figure 4 shows immunohistochemistry with three antibodies at different stages of rat and cat spinal cord development. At E17 Rat 202 stains many axons in the devel-oping spinal cord. Cat 101 recognizes many fewer axons but Cat 201 does not stain the E17 cord. In the rat, Cat 201 first recognizes axons in the third postnatal week. In the cat on postnatal day 1 axons are stained by both Cat 101 and 201 except in the dorsal lateral regions of the spinal cord. In contrast, Rat 202 stains all regions of the P1 spinal cord including the dorsolateral region unstained by Cat 101 and Cat 201. In the adult animal all three antibodies stain axons throughout the white matter of the spinal cord.

The lack of staining in the dorso-lateral region of the spinal cord at P1 may reflect the relatively delayed development of the corticospinal axons (Jones et al. 1982) which run in this region. These results show that axons are not initially found in their fully differentiated state but go through a process of maturation which results in different groups of axons expressing different molecular markers at particular stages of their development.

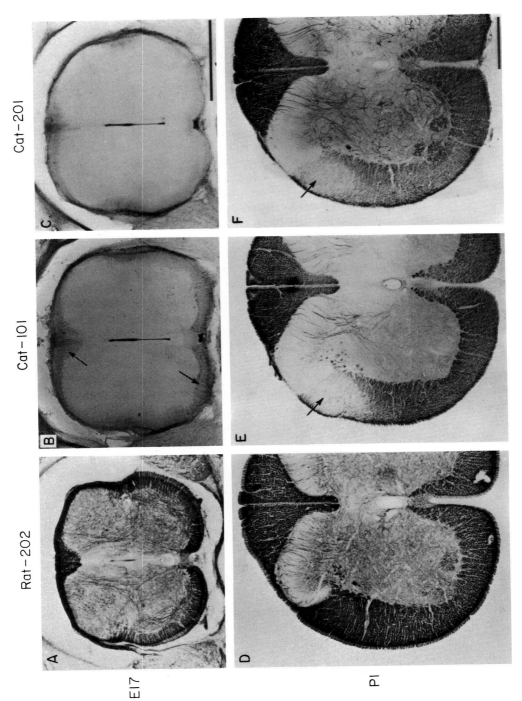

5. Functional and Antigenic Maturation of Neurons in Central Visual Areas

Growing axons in their terminal fields make presynaptic terminals on target cells. The late events of synaptogenesis are strongly influenced by the electrophysiological activity of neurons. Work on the visual system clearly establishes the important role of early visual experience on the anatomical organization and functional capacity of the adult brain (Hubel and Wiesel 1970; Hubel et al. 1977; Wiesel and Hubel 1963a,b, 1965, 1985).

We have shown that hybridomas can be used to reveal unexpected features of the cellular organization of higher visual centers. Monoclonal antibody Cat 301 recognizes a subset of neurons in the lateral geniculate nucleus, the primary visual cortex of cats and primates and in extrastriate visual cortex (Hockfield et al. 1983). In the visual thalamus of cats and primates the antibody Cat 301 recognizes a surface antigen found only around synapses (Hockfield and McKay 1983b) on the soma and proximal dendrites of a subset of neurons. Three lines of evidence show that the Cat 301 positive cells in the lateral geniculate nucleus of the cat are Y cells (Hendry et al. 1984; Hockfield et al. 1985; Sur et al. 1984), a functionally distinct class of neuron (Kalil and Worden 1978; Kratz et al. 1979). (1) The size and location of Cat 301 neurons in the LGN closely corresponds to the distribution of Y cells using anatomical and electrophysiological methods. (2) In the Cat, cortical area 18 receives projections from LGN Y-like cells but not from X cells. In double label experiments 85% of LGN neurons retrogradely labelled by injection of tracer into area 18 are Cat 301 positive. (3) Electrophysiological and anatomical studies have shown that monocular deprivation from birth through a critical postnatal period results in a loss of Y cells. We have examined Cat 301 staining in the LGN of 1-year-old cats monocularly deprived from birth, in these animals there is a dramatic reduction in Cat 301 neurons in the deprived laminae. These results show that the lateral geniculate neurons expressing the Cat 301 antigen are Y cells.

The development of Y cells occurs postnatally in cats and is blocked by the deprivation of light. The expression of the Cat 301 antigen in normal kitten development is coincident with the appearance of Y function and in dark reared or sutured animals the antigen recognized by Cat 301 is absent. These results suggest that late, activity-dependent developmental events lead to neurons acquiring a specific molecular phenotype.

Fig. 4A–F. Developmental maturation of axons. Immunohistochemistry with monoclonal antibodies which identify axonal antigens was carried out on vibratome sections (as in legend to Fig. 1). **A–C** show sections of the E17 rat spinal cord; **D–F** show sections of the P1 cat spinal cord. Different antigenic determinants are expressed at particular times in axon development. A striking example can be seen in **E** and **F** (*arrows*) where the developing cortico-spinal tract is only lightly stained with Cat 101 and Cat 201 even though axons are already present in this region of the neural tube (**D**)

6. Conclusions

A wide range of methods are now used to study differences between cell types in eukaryotes. The studies described in this paper use hybridoma technology to identify both morphologically distinct cell types and specific stages in the differentiation of cell types in the vertebrate central nervous system.

Monoclonal antibody Rat 401 identifies the embryonic radial glial cell. Cells which bind this antibody are initially found in large numbers in the neural tube but during the course of neural development their number declines to zero. The disappearance of antigen positive cells is coincident with the end of the period of neuronal migration. We have also shown that the majority of cells in the G2 phase of the cell cycle are antigen positive throughout neurogenesis. The implication of these findings is that radial glial cells continue to divide during neurogenesis and may be the neural stem cells.

In addition to radial glial cells in the neural tube Rat 401 binds to a cell type found in association with axons throughout the embryo. Antigen positive cells are found in the position of the ventral nerve roots before axons are present. This result suggests that at early times a molecularly distinct non-neuronal cell may lay down axon pathways.

We also summarize evidence showing that as axons mature they express a series of differentiation antigens. Reagents of this kind will be useful in analysing the events which occur as an axon turns from a device for navigation led by a growth cone into an electrically active signalling system ending in a synapse.

Monoclonal antibody Cat 301 has provided a means to follow the postnatal maturation of an electrophysiologically distinct cell type in the dorsal lateral geniculate nucleus of the thalamus, the Y cell. We have shown that this cell type carries a distinct surface antigen associated with a particular set of synapses and that the expression of this antigen is dependent on postnatal visual experience. These results suggest that hybridoma technology may be a powerful tool in the analysis of synaptogenesis during experience-dependent developmental processes.

References

Aguayo AJ, Bray GM, Perkins CM, Duncan D (1979) In: Aspects of developmental biology. Soc Neurosci Symp 4:361–383
Alvarado-Mallart R, Sotelo C (1984) Dev Biol 103:378
Cajal S Ramon (1972) Histologie du Systeme Nerveux Consejo Superior de Investigaciones Cientificas, Instituto Ramon y Cajal, Madrid
Chung SH, Cooke J (1978) Proc R Soc Lond 201:335
Cold Spring Harbor Symp Quant Biol (1983) Vol 48
Dahl D, Rueger D, Bignami A (1981) Eur J Cell Biol 24:191
Galfre G, Howe SC, Milstein C, Butcher GW, Howard JC (1977) Nature 266:550
Harris W (1980) J Comp Neurol 194:303
Hendry SHC, Hockfield S, Jones EG, McKay R (1984) Nature 307:267
Hockfield S, McKay R (1983a) J Neurosci 3:369

Hockfield S, McKay R (1983b) Proc Natl Acad Sci 80:5758

Hockfield S, McKay R (1985) J Neurosci 5:3310

Hockfield S, McKay RD, Hendry SHC, Jones EG (1983) Cold Spring Harbor Symp Quant Biol 48: 877

Hockfield S, Sur M, Frost D, McKay R (1985) Assoc Vision Res Ophthalmol Abstr 26:287

Hubel DH, Wiesel TN (1970) J Physiol 206:419

Hubel DH, Wiesel TN, LeVay S (1977) Phil Trans Rox Soc Lond (B) 278:377

Johansen J, Hockfield S, McKay R (1984) J Comp Neurol 226:263

Jones EG, Schreyer DJ, Wise SP (1982) Prog Brain Res 57:361

Kalil R, Worden I (1978) J Comp Neurol 178:469

Kratz KE, Sherman SM, Kalil R (1979) Science 203:1353

Lance-Jones C, Landmesser L (1980) J Physiol 302:559

Levitt P, Rakic P (1980) J Comp Neurol 193:815

Levitt P, Cooper ML, Rakic P (1981) J Neurosci 1:27

McKay R, Hockfield S (1982) Proc Natl Acad Sci 79:6747

McKay R, Hockfield S, Johansen J, Frederiksen K, Thompson J (1983) Science 222:788

Nordlander RH, Singer JF, Beck R, Singer M (1981) J Comp Neurol 199:535

Ogren MP, McKay R, Schiller PH, Maunsell JHR, Hockfield S (1985) Assoc Vision Res Ophthalmol Abstr 26:163

Rakic P (1971) J Comp Neurol 141:283

Rakic P (1976) Nature 261:467

Rakic P (1981) Trends Neurosci 4:184

Sidman RL (1970) In: Schmitt FO (ed) The neurosciences-second study program. Rockefeller Univ Press, N.Y., pp 100–116

Sidman RL, Miele IL, Fader N (1959) Exp Neurol 1:322

Singer M, Nordlander RH, Egar M (1979) J Comp Neurol 185:1–22

Silver J, Sidman RL (1980) J Comp Neurol 189:101

Spemann H (1938) Embryonic development and induction. Hafner NY

Sur M, Hockfield S, McAvoy M, Garraghty P, Kritzer M, McKay R (1984) Soc Nuurosci Abstr 10: 297

Tapscott S, Bennett G, Toyama Y, Kleinbart F, Holtzer H (1981) Dev Biol 86:40

Vaughn JE, Grieshaber JA (1973) J Comp Neurol 148:177

Wiesel TN, Hubel DH (1963a) J Neurophysiol 26:978

Wiesel TN, Hubel DH (1963b) J Neurophysiol 26:1003

Wiesel TN, Hubel DH (1965) J Neurophysiol 28:1029

Windle WF, Baxter RF (1936) J Comp Neurol 63:189

Zipser B, McKay R (1981) Nature 289:549

The Neural Cell Adhesion Molecule in Development: Examples of Differential Adhesion

U. RUTISHAUSER[1]

1. Introduction

The pioneering studies of Holtfreter (1939) on the contribution of tissue affinities to formation of tissue patterns spurred several decades of work and speculation on the nature of cell-cell interactions. One of the most useful and intriguing concepts to emerge from this period was the potential ability of cells to order themselves according to quantitative differences in adhesiveness (Steinberg 1970), as opposed to the expression of absolute binding specificities. Until recently, too little has been known about the molecular nature of cell-cell adhesion to provide ample evidence that such hierarchies of adhesion actually exist in tissues during their morphogenesis and histogenesis.

Studies over the past decade on the biochemical properties of the neural cell adhesion molecule NCAM (for reviews, see Edelman et al. 1983; Rutishauser 1983) and more recently on the function of NCAM in vivo (see Rutishauser 1984), have provided several examples of how adhesive preferences can contribute to formation of some of the most intricate structures in neural tissue. In this paper these studies are presented primarily in terms of the ability of neurons and growth cones to select targets or pathways according to the adhesive properties of their environment, and then discussed with respect to the differential adhesion hypothesis.

2. The Biochemistry and Expression of NCAM

NCAM is an integral membrane protein with a single polypeptide chain and a large and unusual carbohydrate moiety. For the purposes of this discussion, the key properties of NCAM are (1) that the molecule appears to be a ligand in the formation of cell-cell bonds, (2) that adhesion involves the participation of NCAM molecules on both adhering membranes and therefore is an example of homophilic binding, and (3) that heterogeneity in the carbohydrate moiety can alter the binding properties of the molecule. The last property reflects the content of sialic acid, with a decrease in

---

1 Department of Developmental Genetics and Anatomy, Case Western Reserve University School of Medicine, Cleveland, OH 44106, USA

Molecular Aspects of Neurobiology
(ed. by Rita Levi Montalcini et al.)
© Springer-Verlag Berlin Heidelberg 1986

the length of the unbranched sialic acid chains leading to an *increase* in the apparent binding constant. If NCAM behaves as a homophilic ligand, then cells that express this molecule and come into contact during development have the potential of forming adhesions. The duration and consequences of each adhesion would of course depend on many parameters, two of the most obvious being the concentration and binding affinity of NCAM.

During embryogenesis, NCAM is expressed in a variety of tissues including neuro-epithelia starting with the neural plate, a number of transient structures associated with early morphogenesis such as the notochord, placodes, and somites, and on the three primary cell types found in a differentiated nervous system, that is, neurons, glia, and muscle cells. The focus here will be on the last category and in particular on NCAM-mediated adhesion of neurons to muscle, to glial precursors, and to other neurons.

3. NCAM and Differential Adhesion

At first glance, NCAM seems an unlikely candidate for mediating cell-cell recognition events that lead to the formation of specific tissue structures, in that the molecule has essentially a single binding specificity and a very broad cell and tissue distribution. Recent work, however, has demonstrated that both the expression and form of NCAM are exquisitely regulated in time and space, on individual cells as well as across tissues, in a manner that provides critical opportunities for the choice and timing of appropriate cell-cell interactions. At the level of the cell, the interactions resulting from this regulation appear to involve a simple preference for the most adhesive environment. They therefore represent direct in vivo evidence in support of differential adhesion as a fundamental parameter in histogenesis.

4. Temporal Regulation of NCAM

Two examples have been found in which changes in the expression of NCAM alter adhesive preferences and lead to an important rearrangement of embryonic structures. The first concerns the migration of the neural crest cells destined to become spinal ganglia (Thiery et al. 1982). Prior to their migration, these cells express NCAM and adhere strongly to the dorsal edge of the neural tube. During migration, they appear to no longer have NCAM on their surface, and instead use adhesion to a fibronectin-rich pathway to reach their appropriate site. Upon arrival, they once again express NCAM and are observed to form a compact ganglion.

The second example involves the initial innervation of skeletal muscle by spinal cord neurons. In this case, the NCAM-rich nerve appears to wait at the periphery of the muscle until the latter, by its own internal program, also produces large amounts of the molecule (Tosney et al., in prep.). At that time, the nerve-muscle association becomes more intimate, with extensive ramification of the axon into the muscle, and ultimately results in the formation of electrically active synapses.

Clearly, the temporal aspect of these phenomena lies beyond the immediate scope of the differential adhesion process. What they illustrate, however, is that at the cellular level the effects of the temporal programs are expressed as morphogenetic changes via adhesive preferences for NCAM-containing substrates.

5. Polarity in the Expression of NCAM Across a Cell

When the axons of retinal ganglion cells exit the eye, they follow a stereotyped route along the outer margin of the neuroepithelium, with their growth cones in close apposition to the endfeet of radial glial-like cells. Studies on the expression of NCAM in the neuroepithelium have revealed that the molecule is not only produced by these radial cells, but that its initial distribution, prior to the arrival of axons, is heavily concentrated at their endfeet (Silver and Rutishauser 1984). Such an unusual pattern of expression suggested that the preference of growth cones for endfeet might reflect NCAM-mediated adhesion. This hypothesis was supported by studies showing that antibodies against NCAM alter the route, but not the growth rate of retinal ganglion cell axons. Thus, the growth cones have sufficient adhesion in the absence of NCAM function to promote growth of their axons, but it is the differential adhesivity to NCAM on the endfeet that appears to specify their position at the neuroepithelial margin.

6. Expression of NCAM in Tissue Regions

Optic axons not only grow along the brain margin, but also select a zone of growth that carries them up over the roof of the brain to their ultimate target, the optic tectum. In the same studies cited above (Silver and Rutishauser 1984), it was found that the neuroepithelium restricts NCAM expression to a population of endfeet that constitutes a "pathway" exactly conforming to this growth zone. Again, the pattern of NCAM was present prior to the arrival of optic axon growth cones. With respect to differential affinity, the interpretation of these findings is similar to that given above, that is, the regulation of NCAM, in this case within a sheet of cells, creates a situation in which a relative preference of growth cones for NCAM-mediated adhesion results in part in the specification of a major axonal pathway.

7. Differences in the Structural Form of NCAM

There are a variety of transcriptional and post-translational events that give rise to NCAM molecules with different structures. The chemical heterogeneity that presently appears to be of greatest consequence to differential adhesion is the variability in sialic acid content described above, which can occur both as a function of age and tissue source. The existence of NCAMs that have the same binding specificity but different affinities potentially provides the most dramatic example of differential adhesion. However, it has not as yet been possible to demonstrate clearly that a difference in NCAM sialylation actually results in an adhesive preference during development. The most suggestive evidence is that, at the time when the visual system is formed, the NCAM on optic axons within the eye is of the less-sialylated (more adhesive) form, whereas outside the eye it is of the heavily-sialylated form (Schlosshauer et al. 1984). In terms of adhesive preferences, it has been suggested that the more adhesive form in the eye helps to keep the optic fibers together as they collect into the optic nerve, whereas the less adhesive form allows the axons to begin rearranging themselves and ultimately to choose the appropriate positional cues on the tectal surface. Another recent finding in support of a role for NCAM sialic acid in histogenesis has been that an endoneuraminidase that specifically enhances the adhesiveness of NCAM also causes a number of developmental abnormalities in the eye (Rutishauser et al., in prep.). What is now required to establish further that these observations lead to or represent differential adhesion is a detailed anatomical analysis demonstrating that the perturbation by neuraminidase actually alters membrane-membrane associations.

8. Summary

The concept of differential adhesion was offered originally as a general mechanism for arranging cells in tissues during development (Steinberg 1970). It offered no molecular basis for the adhesive differences except that the sorting out of cells with different affinities *within* an aggregate, rather than into separate aggregates, was taken as evidence that there were hierarchical rather than absolute preferences among the cells. This discussion has summarized relatively direct evidence, with adhesion mediated by a particular molecule, that differential adhesion of the general type proposed by Steinberg actually operates in the embryo. Nevertheless, while such events do seem to occur, they do not by themselves account for histogenesis, but rather represent one of the last and physically most obvious steps in a complex and multi-step process.

Acknowledgments. The work described in this discussion was in part supported by NIH Grant HD 18369.

References

Edelman GM, Hoffman S, Chuong C-M, Thiery J-P, Brackenbury R, Gallin WJ, Grumet M, Greenberg ME, Hemperly JJ, Cohen C, Cunningham BA (1983) Structure and modulation of neural cell adhesion molecules in early and late embryogenesis. Cold Spring Harbor Symp Quant Biol 48:515–526
Holtfreter J (1939) Tissue affinity, a means of embryological morphogenesis. Translated in: Willier B, Oppenheimer J (eds) Foundations in experimental embryology. Prentice-Hall, Englewood Cliffs, NJ (1964), pp 186–225

Rutishauser U (1983) Molecular and biological properties of a neural cell adhesion molecule. Cold
    Spring Harbor Symp Quant Biol 48:501–514
Rutishauser U (1984) Developmental biology of a neural cell adhesion molecule. Nature 310:
    549–554
Rutishauser U, Watanabe M, Silver J, Vimr ER (in prep.) Specific alteration of NCAM-mediated
    cell adhesion by an endoneuraminidase
Schlosshauer B, Schwartz U, Rutishauser U (1984) Topological distribution of different forms of
    NCAM in the developing chick visual system. Nature 310:141–143
Silver J, Rutishauser U (1984) Guidance of optic axons by a preformed adhesive pathway on
    neuroepithelial endfeet. Dev Biol 106:485–499
Steinberg MS (1970) Does differential adhesion govern self assembly processes in histogenesis?
    J Exp Zool 173:395–434
Thiery J-P, Duband J-L, Rutishauser U, Edelman GM (1982) Cell adhesion molecules in early chick
    embryogenesis. Proc Natl Acad Sci 79:6737–6741
Tosney K, Watanabe M, Landmesser L, Rutishauser U (1985) NCAM distribution in the chick hind-
    limb during axon outgrowth and the establishment of mature nerve-muscle relationships.
    Neurosci Abstr (in press)

Molecular Mechanisms of Cell Adhesion in Neurogenesis

J.P. THIERY[1]

1. Introduction

Even in the simplest animals, the neuronal network is extraordinarily intricate. Recent studies have focused on the early development of these highly ordered structures during embryogenesis. Already in 1924, Spemann and Mangold made the remarkable discovery that the neural primordium develops in a limited territory of the ectoderm only if transient interactions occur between the ectoderm and the axial mesoderm during gastrulation; however, more than 50 years later, the molecular mechanism underlying the so-called primary induction has not been deciphered. It is also during gastrulation that the body plan is established through a series of complex morphogenetic movements and cell interactions. The very general question of how the DNA can provide the information necessary for the assembly of three dimensional structures has to be raised. Particularly important in this context is the definition of the molecular repertoire and the mechanisms of regulation at the genetic and epigenetic levels that are involved in the elaboration of such highly ordered cell assemblies. The primary processes of development, i.e., cell division, cell migration, cell adhesion, cell differentiation and cell death have been extensively described during the ontogeny of the nervous system (Cowan 1978). These processes are highly interconnected and, at first glance, it is difficult to sort out the different types of interactions into a flow chart. It is clear, however, that cell adhesion and cell movement must contribute decisively to the animal form. In this arena, two different schools of thought developed in the past. On the one hand it has been proposed that cells recognize each other by specific surface molecules; each cell type, and in the nervous system each nerve process, must carry a unique piece of information allowing the establishment of a precise neuronal network. The chemoaffinity hypothesis in its extreme form was advocated by Sperry (1963) to account for stereotyped pattern of the retinotectal connection both in normal animals and during regeneration. On the other hand, cells could also assemble into tissues under the influence of nonspecific electrical, or Van der Waals', forces. It therefore became necessary to initiate a series of studies which would avoid making assumptions on the degree of specificity required for histogenesis. In 1974, Edelman devised an assay based on the use of antibodies to perturb cell-cell adhesion. This assay

1 Institut d'Embryologie du CNRS et du Collège de France, 94130 Nogent-sur-Marne, France

Molecular Aspects of Neurobiology
(ed. by Rita Levi Montalcini et al.)
© Springer-Verlag Berlin Heidelberg 1986

allowed the detection of cell surface antigen(s) involved in early steps of cell adhesion; using polyspecific antibodies which inhibit in vitro adhesion of neural retinal cells, it was possible to find a source of soluble antigens, a subset of which neutralized the inhibitory activity of these antibodies (Brackenbury et al. 1977). The fractionation of the source of antigens led to the identification of a cell surface protein (Thiery et al. 1977) which has been named the neural cell adhesion molecule, NCAM.

Following the same procedure, another cell adhesion molecule (L-CAM) was isolated from chick liver. NCAM and L-CAM are both cell surface glycoproteins which contain binding domains and act as ligands between cells. Surface glycoproteins similar if not identical to NCAM and L-CAM have been isolated more recently in mammals. In fact, these two molecules are most likely to be present in all vertebrate species (Edelman 1983).

2. Appearance and Distribution of NCAM and L-CAM During Embryogenesis

The localization of these two molecules was performed with monospecific antibodies at the light microscopy level (Edelman et al. 1983). NCAM and L-CAM are already expressed at the surface of most, if not all, cells of the chick blastoderm. During gastrulation cells which egress from the upper layer to provide both the mesoderm and the definitive endoderm lose L-CAM and also become progressively devoid of NCAM. In the area of the upper layer which becomes induced into neural tissues, L-CAM also progressively disappears and is finally restricted in its distribution to the non-induced ectoderm. In contrast, NCAM becomes most predominant in the neural plate. NCAM is also found in the axial mesoderm, particularly in the notochord and during somite formation; NCAMis retained in the dermomyotome and subsequently in the myotome. NCAM is also expressed transiently in many tissues, both in the ectoderm and in the mesoderm, while L-CAM becomes localized in all stable epithelia belonging to the three primary germ layer. In the nervous system, NCAM is found on precursors both of glia and neurons. Later, during the formation of the neuronal network, NCAM is found on neural cell bodies and processes, including the growth cones. At least in birds, NCAM is either not detectable or greatly diminished at the surface of mature glial cells. These immunohistological studies, as well the biochemical analyses of the protein recognized by the anti L-CAM and anti-NCAM antibodies, clearly established that the two cell adhesion molecules are widely distributed in the developing embryo and do not exhibit any tissue or cell specificity.

3. Structure and Mechanism of Action of NCAM and L-CAM

NCAM is a high molecular weight glycoprotein (Edelman 1985a). In fact, two polypeptide chains, of 160 and 130 kd, sharing the same amino-terminal sequence, have been found on the surface of central nervous system neurons. A third polypeptide of

120 kd is also detected, particularly in mammals. All three polypeptides are variably glycosylated. In the embryo, NCAM migrates as a diffuse band on polyacrylamide gels in the 180–250 kd molecular weight range. These embryonic molecules have been shown to carry an unusual amount of sialic acid, most of it being organized as poly-sialic acid linked at three sites in the middle of the polypeptide chain. The binding function is located within the 65 kd amino-terminal region, while a substantial portion of the carboxy terminal region is cytoplasmic. CDNA probes for the NCAM molecules have been obtained using c-DNA libraries cloned in the pBR322 and pUC8 plasmids (Murray et al. 1984). Northern analysis showed the presence of two distinct mRNA species corresponding to the 130 kd and 160 kd polypeptide chains. Similar results have been obtained very recently in mammals. A single gene was detected in Southern blot, therefore implying the existence of a differential splicing mechanism to generate the two mRNA species.

L-CAM is also a transmembrane glycoprotein with a polypeptide chain close to 110 kd with about 15 kd carbohydrate distributed at several sites along the molecule. In contrast to NCAM, L-CAM does not change its molecular weight during develop-ment; this finding is consistent with the detection of one 4 kd mRNA species large enough to code for a 110 kd polypeptide (Gallin et al. 1985). The Southern analysis indicated that possibly one to three genes code for L-CAM; however, these data have been obtained in outbred species, which may carry allelic variants of a single structural gene.

Given the distribution of both CAMs and the results of the in vitro aggregation studies, these molecules are very likely to act through homophilic interactions both in homotypic and heterotypic combination. For instance NCAM can mediate adhesion between neurons or between neurons and muscles. However, L-CAM requires calcium to mediate adhesion in contrast to NCAM, which acts through a calcium-independent mechanism.

4. Primary and Secondary CAMs

As mentioned above, the presence of NCAM on neural precursors and its subsequent restriction to the neuronal lineage must imply that other adhesion molecules ensure the binding between neurons and glial cells. A heterotypic binding assay between glial cells and neurons was devised to identify the putative molecules possessing such func-tions (Grumet et al. 1984). Using the immunologically based assay, a glycoprotein which differs from both L-CAM and NCAM was isolated from brain tissue. The neuron-glia cell adhesion molecule (NgCAM) is also a transmembrane glycoprotein. Three polypeptide chains of approximately 200, 130 and 80 kd are detected on immunoblots. It is not yet known whether the 130 and 80 kd bands are two proteoly-tic fragments of the 200 kd molecule or are separately synthesized. As for NCAM, NgCAM does not require calcium. However, this molecule differs both in its structure and its function from NCAM and should be encoded by a distinct gene. Immuno-histological analysis has revealed that NgCAM is expressed only after neuroblasts have become post-mitotic. NgCAM was not detected on glial cells, at least in birds; neither was it detected on other cells types outside the nervous system. Considering its late apperance and restricted distribution NgCAM was designated as a secondary CAM as compared to the two primary CAMs isolated so far.

5. Role of NCAM and NgCAM in Neural Histogenesis

A series of perturbation experiments both in vitro and in vivo have been performed using neural tissues. In vitro, monovalent antibodies directed against NCAM inhibit the adhesion of individual neural cells. It also prevent the formation of histotypic aggregates and the formation of nerve fascicules. Neural retina explants cannot undergo proper morphogenesis in the presence of these antibodies. When applied at the level of the tectum, retinotectal maps cannot become established until the antibodies have disappeared (Fraser et al. 1984). Antibodies to NgCAM prevent the interaction between neurons and glia. In vivo, using cerebellar slices, the migration of post-mitotic neurons from the external granular layer along the radial Bergman glia is also prevented. Both NCAM and NgCAM must play a major role during the migration of neurons, in the formation of fascicules and in the subsequent interactions between glia and neurons (Edelman 1985b). How, then, can specific connections be achieved with these two molecules?

6. Cell Surface Modulation of CAMs

The theory of cell surface modulation was originally elaborated for lymphocytes. Local as well as global cell surface modulation could operate during morphogenesis (Edelman 1983). Local cell surface modulation of CAMs includes prevalence, changes in surface density of these molecules as well as chemical modifications. In addition, there is now increasing evidence for cis interactions between different CAMs (i.e., NCAM and NgCAM).

The four different types of modulations have considerable influence on the binding strength occurring between adjacent cell surfaces. A thirty-fold increase in the rate of aggregation is observed when the concentration of NCAM at the surface of lipid vesicles is doubled while the transition from embryonic to adult forms of NCAM makes the vesicles aggregate five times faster (Hoffman and Edelman 1983). In vivo, NCAM is not equally distributed on cell bodies, nerve processes and growth cones of different parts of the nervous system. NgCAM has a much more striking asymmetric distribution, appearing only very transiently at the surface of cell bodies but remaining mostly on axons; it is further modulated during myelin assembly (Thiery et al. 1985; Daniloff, Chuong, Levi and Edelman, submitted). The different types of modulation must regulate the dynamics of transient interactions that occur in neural histogenesis.

What is most remarkable is that the transient, but coordinated, expression of CAMs is repeatedly observed in all the different embryonic tissues which have been examined so far. NCAM and L-CAM couples have now been seen, not only in the early stages of neurogenesis, but also in the ontogeny of neurogenic placodes, in the kidney (Thiery et al. 1984) and in the formation of skin feathers (Chuong and Edelman 1985, submitted). It is therefore very likely that genes in control of the expression of the primary CAMs are independent from those governing cytodifferentiation (Edelman 1984).

It is not yet clear, however, whether the differential and often polarized expression of the primary CAM (NCAM) and the secondary CAM (NgCAM) are coordinated and controlled in a similar manner. It should be mentioned that differentiation products such as the microtubule-associated proteins are also assembled in defined compartments of the neurons. The recent availability of cDNA probes for these molecules as well as a better understanding of the cis and trans interactions between CAMs should allow the development of a dynamic model for the establishment of the neuronal network.

It may very well be that this network, as exemplified by recent experiments in the adult monkey is still extremely redundant and therefore does not require a vast repertoire of defined markers (Edelman and Finkel 1984); instead, it could be constructed by selection of the appropriate circuitry that is progressively assembled during ontogeny, in part through the relative efficacy of synapses (Finkel and Edelman 1985).

References

Brackenbury R, Thiery JP, Rutishauser U, Edelman GM (1977) Adhesion among neural cells of the chick embryo. I. An immunological assay for molecules involved in cell-cell binding. J Biol Chem 252:6835–6840

Cowan WM (1978) Aspects of neural development. Int Rev Physiol Neurophysiol III 17:149–191

Edelman GM (1976) Surface modulation in cell recognition and cell growth. Science 192:218–226

Edelman GM (1983) Cell adhesion molecules. Science 219:450–457

Edelman GM (1984) Cell adhesion and morphogenesis: the regulator hypothesis. Proc Natl Acad Sci 81:1460–1464

Edelman GM (1985a) Cell adhesion and the molecular processes of morphogenesis. Annu Rev Biochem 54:135–169

Edelman GM (1985b) Cell adhesion molecules in neural histogenesis. Annu Rev Physiol (in press)

Edelman GM, Finkel LH (1984) Neuronal group selection in the cerebral cortex. In: Edelman GM, Cowan WM, Gall WE (eds) Dynamic aspects of neo-cortical function. John Wiley, New York, pp 653–695

Edelman GM, Gallin WJ, Delouvee A, Cunningham BA, Thiery JP (1983) Early epochal maps of two different cell adhesion molecules. Proc Natl Acad Sci 80:4384–4388

Finkel LH, Edelman GM (1985) Interaction of synaptic modification rules within populations of neurons. Proc Natl Acad Sci 82:1291–1295

Fraser SE, Murray BA, Cheng-Ming Chuong, Edelman GM (1984) Alteration of the retinotectal map in Xenopus by antibodies to neural cell adhesion molecules. Proc Natl Acad Sci 81:4222–4226

Gallin WJ, Prediger E, Edelman GM, Cunningham BA (1985) Isolation of a cDNA clone for the liver cell adhesion molecule (L-CAM). Proc Natl Acad Sci 82:2809–2813

Grumet M, Hoffman S, Cheng Ming Chuong, Edelman GM (1984) Polypeptide components and binding functions of neuron-glia cell adhesion molecules. Proc Natl Acad Sci 81:7989–7993

Hoffman S, Edelman GM (1983) Kinetics of homophilic binding by embryonic and adult forms of the neural cell adhesion molecule. Proc Natl Acad Sci UDA 80:5762–5766

Murray BA, Hemperly JJ, Gallin WJ, Mac Gregor JS, Edelman GM, Cunningham BA (1984) Isolation of cDNA clones for the chicken neural cell adhesion molecule (N-CAM). Proc Natl Acad Sci USA 81:5584–5588

Sperry RW (1963) Chemoaffinity in the order by growth of nerve fiber patterns and connections. Proc Natl Acad Sci USA 50:703–710

Thiery JP, Brackenbury R, Rutishauser U, Edelman GM (1977) Adhesion among neural cells of the chick embryo. II Purification and characterization of a cell adhesion molecule from neural retina. J Biol Chem 252:6841–6845

Thiery JP, Delouvee A, Gallin WJ, Cunningham BA, Edelman GM (1984) Ontogenetic expression of cell adhesion molecules: L-CAM is found in epithelia derived from the three primary germ layers. Dev Biol 102:61–78

Thiery JP, Delouvee A, Grumet M, Edelman GM (1985) Initial appearance and regional distribution of the neuron-glia cell adhesion molecule. J Cell Biol 100:442–456

Radial Organization of the Cerebral Cortex: Genetic and Phylogenetic Determinants

A. GOFFINET and C. DAUMERIE[1]

1. Introduction

The mammalian cerebral cortex is characterized by a radial organization which derives from the radial neuronal architectonics of the embryonic cortical plate. This normal cell pattern of the embryonic cortex is necessary for the development of cortical lamination and foliation as well as columnar organization. The purpose of this work is to show that radial organization of the embryonic cortical plate is: (1) the result of a progressive build-up during brain evolution and (2) under genetic control, particularly from the reeler locus (in mice).

2. Radial Cortical Architectonics as an Evolutionary Acquisition

Among vertebrates, mammals and to a lesser extent reptiles have a well developed cerebral cortex. Comparative studies of the embryonic cortex (cortical plate) in the four reptilian radiations and in mammals show that the radial pattern is not uniformly present in all species (Figs. 1 and 2). It is best developed in mammals and squamates, particularly lacertilians, but most rudimentary in turtles, which are considered the most closely related to mammalian ancestors (Northcutt 1981). The organization of the embryonic cortex in other reptilian orders such as crocodilians and *Sphenodon* can be described as intermediate (Goffinet 1983, 1984a). Tritiated thymidine studies of histogenesis in the reptile cortex reveal that earliest generated cells are found closest to the pial surface. That is, the histogenetic gradient is directed from outside to inside (Goffinet et al. 1985). This is in contrast to the mammalian cortex, in which histogenesis proceeds from inside to outside (Caviness and Rakic 1978).

These comparative embryological data show that the radial organization of cortical neurons has been acquired to various extents by vertebrate phyla after their point of divergence. It is an example of homoplasy, resulting from evolutionary convergence. In the reptilian radiation leading to mammals (Fig. 2), radial organization and inside-out histogenetic gradient have appeared in that order. Possibly, radial organization is requisite to the appearance of the inside-out vector of cortical development (vide infra).

---

1 University Louvain Medical School, B–1200 Brussels, Belgium

Molecular Aspects of Neurobiology
(ed. by Rita Levi Montalcini et al.)
© Springer-Verlag Berlin Heidelberg 1986

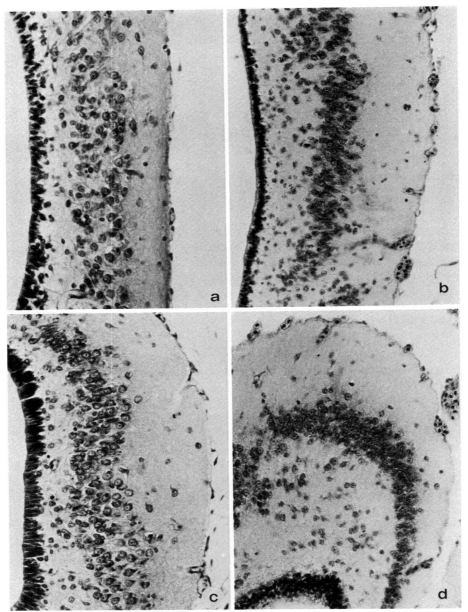

Fig. 1a–d. Comparison of radial architectonics in turtle (a,c) and lizard (b,d), at the level of the dorsal cortex (a,b) and hippocampus (c,d). (×255)

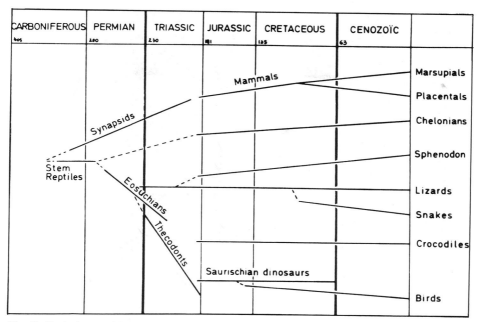

Fig. 2. Evolutionary filiations leading to living reptiles, mammals and birds. Time in millions of years

3. Genetic Control of Radial Cortical Organization: the Reeler Locus in Mice

Reeler (rl) is an autosomal recessive mutation in mice (chromosome 5) which results in a disorganization of architectonic patterns in the central nervous system of homozygous animals (Caviness and Rakic 1978; Goffinet 1984b). From its earliest stage of development, the reeler cortical plate has a defective organization (Fig. 3). The defect is architectonic-selective in that cell-proliferation, extracortical migration, synaptogenesis. . . etc remain relatively unaffected (Caviness 1982; Pinto-Lord et al. 1982). Tritiated thymidine analysis of cortical development in reeler (Caviness 1982) shows that the vector of cortical histogenesis is reversed compared to that in normal animals. That is, cortical development in reeler proceeds from outside to inside as it does in reptiles. This observation suggests that the radial organization of the cortical plate is necessary for the normal (inside-out) development of the mammalian cortex.

Two non-complementing, presumably allelic reeler mutations are known. Phenocopies of the reeler trait have never been observed, neither as the result of mutations at other loci nor following environmental interferences. It follows that the reeler locus can be viewed as a key component in the control of cortical development.

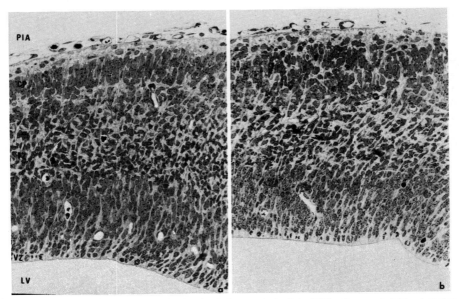

Fig. 3 a,b. Frontal sections at the level of the cortical plate (*CP*) of normal (a) and reeler (b) embryos, at gestational day 14. Note disorganization of the reeler *CP*. (×340)

4. Mechanisms Responsible for Radial Organization of the Embryonic Cortex

Both genetic and phylogenetic data point to the importance of radial organization of embryonic cortical neurons during normal cortical development, and to the role of the reeler locus in this process. Among several mechanisms which could account for cell patterns in the cortical plate, various observations (reviewed by Goffinet 1984b) suggest that local cell-cell interactions are particularly worth considering. These interactions could be homotypic (neuronal-neuronal), heterotypic (glial-neuronal) or both. Recent work on cell surface molecules implicated in cell recognition-adhesion events (e.g. Edelman 1984) suggests that components responsible for the early architectonic organization might be identified in the near future. The elucidation of mechanisms involved, particularly of the action of the reeler gene, would represent a significant progress in our understanding of brain development.

References

Caviness VS Jr (1982) Neocortical histogenesis in normal and reeler mice: a developmental study based upon H-3-Thymidine autoradiography. Dev Brain Res 4:293–302

Caviness VS Jr, Rakic P (1978) Mechanisms of cortical development: a view from mutations in mice. Annu Rev Neurosci 1:297–326

Edelman GM (1984) Modulation of cell adhesion during induction, histogenesis and perinatal development of the nervous system. Annu Rev Neurosci 7:339–378

Goffinet AM (1983) The embryonic development of the cortical plate in reptiles. J Comp Neurol 215:437–452

Goffinet AM (1984a) Phylogenetic determinants of radial organization in the cerebral cortex. Z Mikrosk-Anat Forsch 98:909–925

Goffinet AM (1984b) Events governing organization of postmigratory neurons: studies on brain development in normal and reeler mice. Brain Res Rev 7:261–296

Goffinet AM, Daumerie Ch, Langerwerf B, Pieau C (1985) Neurogenesis in the reptile cortex: H-3-Thymidine autoradiographci analysis. Soc Neurosci Abstr (in press)

Northcutt RG (1981) Evolution of the telencephalon in non mammals. Annu Rev Neurosci 4: 301–350

Pinto-Lord MC, Evrard Ph, Caviness VS Jr (1982) Obstructed neuronal migration along radial glial fibers in the neocortex of the reeler mouse: a Golgi-EM analysis. Dev Brain Res 4:379–393

Regulation of Dorsal Root Ganglia Proteins and Genes During Early Development and Synaptogenesis

M.C. FISHMAN, S.-C. NG, K. WOOD, and L. BAIZER[1]

1. Introduction

Neurons of the dorsal root ganglia derive from neural crest precursor cells. Shortly after arrival of neural crest precursors to the coalescing ganglia, neurons are "born" as the cells undergo their final mitosis, generating first the large and then small diameter populations of DRG neurons. By about embryonic day 15 these neurons have extended processes to the spinal cord. The first evidence for synaptic interaction between dorsal root ganglia and spinal cord neurons begins about embryonic day 17. Significant maturation of the synapses occurs subsequently and continues through birth, with progressively larger areas of synaptic contact and increased numbers of presynaptic vesicles (Lawson et al. 1974). We have been interested in determining the molecules involved in these transitions, as neuronal precursor becomes post-mitotic neuron, and then as it ceases growth cone exploration and makes stable and specific synapses. We have used two techniques to isolate such molecules. First, we have determined proteins transported to synaptic regions prior to and after synapse formation. Second, we have established cDNA libraries from critical stages during development and have compared gene expression using the technique of differential hybridization to search for stage-specific cDNA's. We have been especially interested in those molecules that characterize precursor and early embryonic states and diminish during maturation.

2. Methods

2.1 Axonally Transported Proteins

Dorsal root ganglia of embryonic day 17 rats were dissected and plated as described previously (Sonderegger et al. 1983). Compartmental cell culture chambers were utilized to provide separation of soma and growing axons, chambers in which soma were restricted to the center compartment while their axons extend to the sides. Electrical recording revealed that target spinal cord cells in the side compartment were

---

1 Massachusetts General Hospital, Harvard Medical School, Boston, MA 02114, USA

innervated by DRG cells in the center. Axonally transported proteins were metabolically labeled in the presence or absence of target cells and then displayed on two-dimensional polyacrylamide gels.

2.2 cDNA Cloning

About 10,000 dorsal root ganglia were harvested from rats at embryonic day 13, embryonic day 17 and postnatal days 3–4. mRNA was isolated by standard procedures and cDNA generated and inserted into the EcoR1 site of the vectors lambda gt10 and lambda gt11. Cloning efficiencies of about 10^6 plaques per microgram poly(A)$^+$RNA were obtained. In vitro translation was performed using reticulocyte lysate. Differential screening of each library was performed using radioactive cDNAs.

3. Results

3.1 Axonally Transported Proteins

The two-dimensional gel profile of cultured dorsal root ganglia neurons included about 300 distinct proteins. This profile was not noticeably different when target cells were provided to the axons. A subcategory of these DRG proteins was transported to the axons. Using chick dorsal root ganglia, four axonally transported proteins were identified that changed in concentration in the presence of target cells. Two proteins, with apparent molecular weights (mol.wt.) of 65,000 and 50,000, both diminished, and two proteins of mol.wt. about 60,000 increased (Sonderegger et al. 1983). This target regulation of presynaptic proteins was exerted only by the presence of the target cells and not by conditioned medium. However, the magnitude of these changes was small, perhaps because not all presynaptic axons contacted appropriate target neurons.

More recently, using rat dorsal root ganglia we have identified a higher molecular weight axonal protein of about mol.wt. 210,000 that diminishes when target cells are contacted. Axonally transported proteins can be further characterized into rapid and slow components, the former including glycoproteins presumably destined for membrane insertion (Tytell et al. 1981) and the latter including cytoskeletal components such as actin and tubulin. The 210K protein is rapidly transported but does not appear to be an integral membrane protein. This protein seems rather to be secreted by the DRG neuron. Its relative level diminishes when target cells are contacted but at present it is not clear that this control is restricted to specific target neurons. Contact with non-neuronal cells of the dorsal root ganglia do not, however, affect its concentration. This axonally transported and secreted protein is of interest in light of recent evidence for the contribution of presynaptic proteins to the extracellular space at the synapse (Caroni et al. 1985).

3.2 cDNA Cloning

mRNA was isolated from different stages, translated in vitro, and displayed on two-dimensional gels. Several of the translated proteins appeared to be stage-specific. Most markedly two basic translation products with mol.wt. of about 10,000 diminished from day 13 to day 17. One of these disappeared completely by postnatal day 3. Several of the translation products appeared to increase concomitantly. This suggests that there are developmentally regulated changes even in the relatively abundant mRNA populations at these particular stages. Thus, we have constructed cDNA libraries in lambda gt10 and lambda gt11. Preliminary differential screening has identified clones in the E13 library labeled in an apparent stage-specific manner.

4. Discussion

These particular gene products are candidates for molecules involved in the cellular transitions of the embryonic neurons. Thus, as the cells relinguish their mitotic and migratory neural crest character it is not unreasonable to expect changes in gene expression, as we have found. Similarly, the observed changes in the population of axonally transported molecules may reflect the maturation from growth cone to synapse. It is clear that some molecules of the DRG will increase in abundance during this period, such as those related to synaptic transmission. Thus, mRNA for somatostatin in the DRG increases only after birth (Fishman and Zingg, unpubl.) and immunoreactive substance P levels increase during later embryogenesis (Schwartz and Costa 1979). However, it will also be of interest to investigate the nature of control over the mRNA species and axonally transported proteins that we have identified that preferentially characterize precursor stages and diminish during development.

References

Caroni P, Carlson SS, Schweitzer E, Kelly RB (1985) Presynaptic neurones may contribute a unique glycoprotein to the extracellular matrix at the synapse. Nature 314:441–443
Lawson SN, Caddy KWT, Biscoe TJ (1974) Development of rat dorsal root ganglion neurons: Studies in cell birthdays and changes in mean cell diameter. Cell Tissue Res 153:399–413
Schwartz JP, Costa E (1979) Nerve growth factormediated increase of the substance P content of chick embryo dosal root ganglia. Brain Res 170:198–202
Sonderegger P, Fishman MC, Bokoum M, Bauer MC, Nelson PG (1983) Axonal proteins of presynaptic neurons during synaptogenesis. Science 221:1294–1297
Tytell M, Black MM, Garner JA, Lasek RJ (1981) Axonal transport: each major rate component reflects the movement of distinct macromolecular complexes. Science 214:179–181

Astrocytic Cell Clones from Mouse Cerebella Induce Differentiation of Embryonic Neuroblasts

B. PESSAC and F. ALLIOT[1]

Two roles have been proposed for astroglia in establishing the cellular architecture of the developing mammalian cerebellum. First, radially oriented astroglial processes are thought to guide the migration of immature granule cells from the pial surface (ventricular zone), where they undergo their final mitosis to the internal granular layer where they form synaptic connections (Rakic 1971). Second, after neuronal migration, protoplasmic astrocytes organize mature granule cells into compartments (Palay and Chan-Palay 1974). The aim of the present work was to search for a role of astroglial cells in differentiation of the neuroblasts of the cerebellum. This requires the development of a tissue culture system where interactions between the different types of astrocytes and neuroblasts can be studied. The method we have chosen to obtain adequate quantities of homogenous astrocytes is the derivation of permanent clonal cells with astroglial properties from explant cultures of 8-day post-natal C57Bl mouse cerebella. These cultures acquired "spontaneously", i.e. without addition of either carcinogens or oncogenic viruses, the capacity to develop into permanent cell lines from which many clones have been derived. Some of these clones synthesize GFAP, a property characteristic of astroglial cells; in addition they do not bind tetanus toxin or the monoclonal antibody A2B5 and they have no oligodendroglial marker such as surface galactocerebroside or myelin basic protein. These cerebellar astroglial clones can be distinguished according to their morphology into three separate types that may represent the Golgi epithelial cells and their Bergmann fibers, the fibrous and the velate protoplasmic astrocytes (Alliot and Pessac 1984).

We have asked the question whether these astrocytic cells clones could have a distinct effect on the differentiation of neuroblasts from 14-day embryonic mouse cerebella. At that stage the only neurons that are about to complete their last round of mitosis are Purkinje, Golgi and deep nuclei cells. The experimental protocol consists in seeding suspensions of single cells upon "monolayers" of each of these clones. The cell suspensions adhere readily and equally well to the three astrocytic clones as 80–90% of the cells are firmly attached after 3 h. Among them, the neuroblasts and neurons are identified by their binding of tetanus toxin as demonstrated by the indirect immunofluorescence technique. They represent about 2/3 of the cell population. The embryonic neurons survive well on the Golgi epithelial-like cells and on the

---

1 INSERM U178, Bât. INSERM, 16 av. P.V. Couturier, 94807 Villejuif Cedex, France

Molecular Aspects of Neurobiology
(ed. by Rita Levi Montalcini et al.)
© Springer-Verlag Berlin Heidelberg 1986

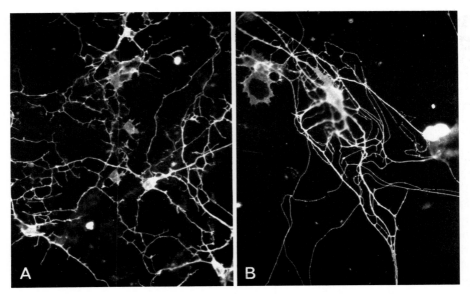

Fig. 1 A,B. Cocultures of cell suspensions from 15-day mouse embryonic cerebella upon layers of astrocytic clones. The neurons are visualized after 6 days by tetanus toxin binding (indirect immunofluorescence technique). **A** Golgi epithelial-like cells. **B** Protoplasmic-like cells. (×255)

protoplasmic-like astrocytes as their number remains roughly constant during the first week of culture; while at that time very few neurons are present on the fibrous-like astrocytes.

The neuroblasts cocultured on each of the astrocytic cell clones differentiate with a distinct pattern. First, starting after 2 days, the morphology of the neuroblasts depends on the astrocytic layer on which they are cocultured. On the Golgi epithelial-like astrocytes, most neurons have few long thin highly branched and sinuous processes (Fig. 1A). On the protoplasmic-like astrocytes, the majority of neurons have small somas, are bipolar, extend long, straight, thick, bifurcated processes which give rise to recurrent branches with a spiderweb-like morphology (Fig. 1B). During the first days of culture on the fibrous-like astrocytes many neurons are flat and the processes present on some cells were short and unbranched. Also the neuroblasts seeded on fibroblasts monolayers aggregated rapidly and appeared poorly differentiated.

The capacity to synthesize GABA, one of the major neurotransmitters of cerebellum neurons, was also investigated. The presence of GABA was detected with monospecific anti-GABA antisera provided by M. Geffard (Seguela et al. 1984) and A. Towbie. After 24 h of culture on either type of astrocytic clone, GABA is present in 25 35% of the embryonic neurons. A few days later, however, there are twice as many GABA positive neurons on the protoplasmic astrocytes (Fig. 2), than on the Golgi epithelial cells.

In order to identify the various types of neurons that differentiate from the embryonic neuroblasts cocultured with the astroglial clones, we have begun to use monoclonal antibodies that appear to recognize distinct cell types. We have used the mono-

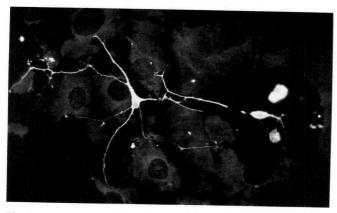

Fig. 2. GABA immunoreactivity in cerebellar embryonic neurons cultured on a layer of protoplasmic astrocytes. (×255)

clonal antibodies 7-8-D2 and 8-20-1 that appear specific for rat (Webb and Woodhams 1984) and mouse (unpubl. data) granule cells in primary cultures of 8-day post-natal cerebellum. Our preliminary results indicate that about 50% of the embryonic neuroblasts acquire the 7-8-D2 and 8-20-1 epitopes after a few days of coculture on the protoplasmic astrocytes.

Taken together these data show that monolayers of Golgi epithelial-like and protoplasmic-like astrocytes permit the survival of embryonic cerebella neurons and each induce a distinct neuronal differentiation pattern.

References

Alliot F, Pessac B (1984) Astrocytic cell clones derived from established cultures of 8-day post-natal mouse cerebella. Brain Res 306:283–291

Palay SL, Chan-Palay V (eds) (1974) In: Cerebellar cortex. Cytology and organization. Springer, Berlin Heidelberg New York

Rakic P (1971) Neuron-glia relationship during granule cell migration in developing cerebellar cortex. A Golgi and electron microscopic study in *Macacus Rhesus*. J Comp Neurol 141:282–312

Seguela P, Geffard M, Muijs RM, Le Moal M (1984) Antibodies against γ-aminobutyric acid: specificity studies and immunocytochemical results. Proc Natl Acad Sci USA 81:3888–3891

Webb M, Woodhams PL (1984) Monoclonal antibodies recognizing cell surface molecules expressed by rat cerebellar interneurones. J Neuroimmunol 6:283–300

Cell Interactions in the Morphogenesis of the Neural Crest

D.F. NEWGREEN[1]

1. Introduction

The neural crest of vertebrate embryos is formed by epithelial cells lying between the neural plate ectoderm and the more lateral epidermal ectoderm. As the neural plate folds to form the neural tube, the neural crest is brought to a dorso-medial position. At around this stage the neural crest population starts to transform from an epithelium to mesenchyme. These mesenchymal cells then disperse, initially into adjacent spaces filled with extracellular matrix (ECM). In the following stages, the cells of this lineage localize at discrete, often distant sites where overt differentiation takes place (see Le Douarin 1982). The orderly execution of this complex pattern of morphogenesis clearly rests on an interaction of these cell with their cellular and non-cellular environment. Some of the interactions that control the development of this system are discussed below, using the avian embryo as a model.

2. The Onset of Neural Crest Cell Dispersion

Precocious dispersion of neural crest cell could be prevented by physical blockade (e.g. by basal laminae, or insufficient space), by unfavourable surroundings (e.g. by inadequate ECM substrates), by inherent locomotory incompetence (e.g. by inactivity of filopodia, or lack of receptors for substrate molecules), or by restraining cell-cell adhesions. Dispersion would occur on the change of these preventive conditions to permissive: the timetable would be controlled by the last to change. Other than cell-cell adhesions, all these conditions seem to be permissive prior to the onset of dispersion as judged by electron microscopy (Newgreen and Gibbins 1982). When tested functionally in vitro, the adhesion of neural crest cells to cells of the neural anlage remained high until the normal time of onset of dispersion, then declined markedly (Newgreen and Gibbins 1982). Inactivation of Ca^{2+}-dependent adhesions by protease in the absence of Ca^{2+} (see Takeichi et al. 1979) caused a precocious disaggregation of cells and consequent premature dispersion of neural crest cells (Newgreen and Gooday

---

1 Abteilung Biochemie, Max-Planck-Institut für Entwicklungsbiologie, D–7400 Tübingen, FRG

Molecular Aspects of Neurobiology
(ed. by Rita Levi Montalcini et al.)
© Springer-Verlag Berlin Heidelberg 1986

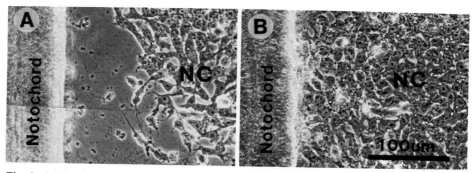

Fig. 1. A Neural crest cells (*NC*) growing in vitro on ECM are unable to approach a co-cultured *Notochord*. B Inclusion of chondroitinase ABC (1.5 U/ml) enables neural crest cells to occupy ECM adjacent to the *Notochord*. Phase contrast

1985). On the other hand, immunolabeling showed that the Ca^{2+}-independent adhesive molecule NCAM was also reduced on neural crest cells around the time of onset of dispersion (Thiery et al. 1982). Thus at least two cell-cell adhesion system decrease on neural crest cells: this very likely controls the time-table of onset of dispersion in aves.

3. The Routes of Neural Crest Cell Dispersion

Neural crest cell dispersion is restricted (at least initially) to cell-free spaces, but not all spaces are equally followed by the cells. Beyond some minimal requirement, the actual dimensions of these spaces are not a limiting factor on dispersion (Anderson and Meier 1982). The ECM components of these spaces may, however, determine their suitability for neural crest cells. Immunoreactivity for fibronectin (Newgreen and Thiery 1980) laminin, collagen (types I to IV), vitronectin and chondroitin-6-sulphate proteoglycan (U. Gaul and D. Newgreen, unpublished) have been found in the ECM. When tested in vitro, fibronectin, laminin (Newgreen 1984) and vitronectin strongly favored neural crest cell adhesion and translocation, compared to collagen (Newgreen et al. 1982). In contrast, a chondroitin sulphate proteoglycan had an antagonistic effect (Newgreen 1982). Moreover, chondroitinase ABC-sensitive, *Streptomyces* hyaluronidase-resistant ECM released by the notochord can prevent neural crest cells from moving on complex ECM in culture (Fig. 1). Detailed study of the distribution of proteoglycan stained for TEM with ruthenium red showed that neural crest cells in vivo don't enter areas with densest proteoglycan (Newgreen et al. 1982). These in vivo and in vitro observations indicate that neural crest cell distribution is in part governed by adhesive interactions with the ECM, which in turn involve a balance between fibronectin (and possibly other favorable macromolecules) and chondroitin sulphate proteoglycan.

Table 1. Extension of cells and axons from explants of quail embryo tissue

Explant	Donor Age (days)	Outgrowth	Substrate				
			CEF + ECM	ECM	FN	LN	Coll. gel
NA	2	NCC	0/+	+++	+++	+++	++
Feather	8–9	Mel	+++	+/++	0	0	0
DRG	8–9	Axon	++	+	+	+++	+
SyG	8–9	Axon	++	+	+	+++	+

Abbreviations: NA, neural anlage; DRG, dorsal root ganglion; SyG, sympathetic ganglion; NCC, neural crest cell; Mel, melanocyte; CEF, chick embryo fibroblast; ECM, fibroblastic extracellular matrix; FN, fibronectin; LN, laminin; Coll., collagen type I

4. The Localization of Neural Crest Cells

The cessation of dispersion of neural crest cells could be influenced by changes in the cells' responses to their surroundings. When tested in vitro thoraco-lumbar neural crest cells, isolated during the dispersive phase showed different preferences for extension on different substrates. Likewise, the extension ability of derivatives of these cells isolated after cessation of dispersion, varied with the substrate, but the order of preference was altered. Neural crest cells extended equally well on fibronectin-rich ECM, fibronectin and laminin, and were retarded on fibroblasts plus ECM. In contrast, neural crest-derived melanocytes from feather explants spread preferentially on fibroblasts plus ECM, in comparison with ECM alone, whereas fibronectin, laminin and collagen gels could not elicit outgrowth. Outgrowth of axons from neural crest-derived ganglia occurred preferentially on laminin in comparison with other substrates tested (Table 1). From these results, it is obvious that the affinity of neural crest cells for elements of their environment changes as they differentiate, and this varies with the line of differentiation. Changes of this nature could contribute to the control of the distribution of neural crest cells as they pass from the dispersive to the localization phase.

References

Anderson CB, Meier S (1982) Effect of hyaluronidase treatment on the distribution of cranial neural crest cells in the chick embryo. J Exp Zool 221:329–335

Le Douarin NM (1982) The neural crest. Cambridge University Press, Cambridge

Newgreen DF (1982) Adhesion to extracellular materials by neural crest cells at the stage of initial migration. Cell Tissue Res 227:297–317

Newgreen DF (1984) Spreading of explants of embryonic chick mesenchymes and epithelia on fibronectin and laminin. Cell Tissue Res 236:265–277

Newgreen DF, Gibbins I (1982) Factors controlling the time of onset of the migration of neural crest cells in the fowl embryo. Cell Tissue Res 224:145–160

Newgreen DF, Gooday D (1985) Control of the onset of migration of neural crest cells in avian embryos. Role of Ca^{2+}-dependent cell adhesions. Cell Tissue Res 239:329–336

Newgreen DF, Thiery JP (1980) Fibronectin in early avian embryos: Synthesis and distribution along migration pathways of neural crest cells. Cell Tissue Res 221:269–291

Newgreen DF, Gibbins IL, Sauter J, Wallenfels B, Wutz R (1982) Ultrastructural and tissue culture studies on the role of fibronectin, collagen and glycosaminoglycans in the migration of neural crest cells in the fowl embryo. Cell Tissue Res 221:521–549

Takeichi M, Ozaki HS, Tokunaga K, Okada TS (1979) Experimental manipulations of cell surface to affect cellular recognition mechanisms. Dev Biol 70:195–205

Thiery JP, Duband JL, Rutishauser U, Edelman GM (1982) Cell adhesion molecules in early chicken morphogenesis. Proc Natl Acad Sci USA 79:6737–6741

Persistent Rabies Virus Infection of Neuronal Cells Causes Defects in Neuroreceptor Regulation

K. KOSCHEL, P. MÜNZEL, M. HALBACH, and R. METZNER [1]

1. General Aspects

Some neurological diseases in man or animals are caused by neurotropic viruses which infect brain cells acutely or persistently. The relationship between virus infection and impairments of neural functions is difficult to clarify biochemically in vivo. Therefore we used CNS-derived permanent cell lines with defined neurobiochemical properties. Such cells can be acutely or persistently infected by viruses. Acute infections will kill the cells whereas persistent infections do not influence general cell parameters such as growth and cell morphology. The question we asked was: Is there an influence of persistent virus infection on specialized neurobiochemical functions. It is quite clear that impairments of these functions would cause disturbances and disorders in the brain without destruction of cells.

2. 108CC15 Cells and Rabies Virus

One of the CNS-derived permanent cell lines used in our studies were the neuron-like mouse neuroblastoma-rat glioma cell hybrids 108CC15 (resp. NG 108-15) (see Hamprecht 1977 for review). These cells show different neurohormone and neurotransmitter receptors, can differentiate into cholinergic cells, can form synapses together with skeletal muscle cells and show electrical excitability. The hybrid cells could be infected by rabies virus either acutely or persistently. The latter type of infection would allow the study of the impairment of specialized cellular functions. Such a specialized function, for example, is the regulation of the cAMP level via membrane receptors: PGE_1 stimulate via PGE_1-receptors the cAMP synthesis and opiates inhibit this stimulation via δ-type opiate receptors (Fig. 1A).

---

1 Institut für Virologie und Immunbiologie der Universität Würzburg, Versbacher Straße 7, D−8700 Würzburg, FRG

Molecular Aspects of Neurobiology
(ed. by Rita Levi Montalcini et al.)
© Springer-Verlag Berlin Heidelberg 1986

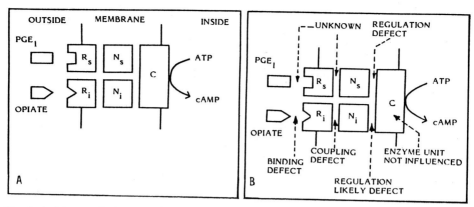

Fig. 1. A Scheme of PGE$_1$ recrptor/adenylate cyclase system, counteracted by the opiate receptor system in 108CC15 cells. **B** Impairments of the system in persistently rabiesvirus infected 108CC15 cells. R_s PGE$_1$ receptor; R_i opiate receptor; C catalytic cyclase unit; N_S stimulating GTP binding regulatory protein; N_i inhibiting GTP binding regulatory protein

The following results were obtained in rabies virus infected cells:

1. A strong inhibition (about 50%) of the PGE$_1$ stimulated cAMP synthesis in intact cells (Koschel and Halbach 1979).
2. Plasma membrane fractions of such persistently infected cells show an inhibition of the function of the stimulating regulatory GTP binding protein N$_S$ of the adenylate cyclase system: The N$_S$ unit does not stimulate the catalytic cyclase unit. The cyclase unit however is fully active using forskoline as direct activator of this unit (Koschel and Münzel 1984).
3. In the persistently infected cells we observed a total loss of the opiate receptor function: Opiates do not inhibit the PGE$_1$-induced increase of cAMP synthesis (Halbach and Koschel 1979).

This loss of opiate receptor function was analyzed in more details (a) by receptor binding of the agonist ^{2}H-etorphine to cell membrane preparations and (b) by studying the opiate receptor coupling to the inhibiting regulatory GTP binding protein N$_i$. We obtained the following results:

4. Binding of agonists on membranes of acutely and persistently infected cells have shown a drastic decrease of binding constants in comparison with membranes of uninfected cells (acutely infected 10-fold, persistently infected 20-fold) without changes of the number of receptors (Münzel and Koschel 1981).

This change of binding affinity however cannot be the reason for the loss of opiate receptor function since very high concentrations of opiates cannot overcome the loss of inhibiting function. Further research showed another important defect:

5. Persistently infected cells are unable to couple the opiate receptor to the inhibiting regulatory protein N$_i$, measured by the opiate stimulated GTPase activity of this N$_i$ unit (Koschel and Münzel 1984).

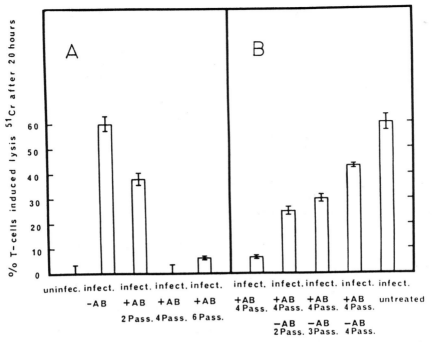

Fig. 2A,B. Antigenic modulation of viral antigens by human antiviral antibodies and cytotoxic T-cell lysis of persistently rabies virus infected 108CC15 cells (C3H mouse neuroblastoma-rat glioma). Spleen lymphocytes from rabies virus antigen (purified, Pasteur Insitute, Paris) immunized C3H mice were used as effector cells (effector cells:target cells = 50:1). Cytotoxic lysis was measured after 1.5 h incubation by release of ^{51}Chromium from ^{51}Cr prelabeled target cells. **A** Down modulation and cytotoxic lysis. *AB* antiviral antibodies (50 hemagglutination inhibiting units); *Pass* passages (every second day). **B** Reversion of antigenic down modulation after removal of *AB* and cytotoxic lysis

Neither high concentrations of GTP nor high concentrations of opiate can overcome this defect. A summary of the results is given in Fig. 1B.

3. Immune System and Persistent Virus Infection

Some important questions arise which are connected to the immune response in the CNS:

1. How can a cytopathic virus establish a persistent infection in the CNS and what is the role of the immune system in this process?
2. Why are infected cells in the CNS not eliminated by immune responses?
3. Why do persistently infected cells in the CNS not show disorders of their functions for a long time?
4. What controls the change from the "silent" state of persistence to a dramatic development of a fatal disease accompanied by cell destruction?

The key role of the immune system in the above questions is the observation of Fujinami and Oldstone (1980) and ourselves (Barret and Koschel 1983) that viral antigens can be modulated by antiviral antibodies recognizing viral hemagglutinine on the cell surface. Growing persistently infected cells for some passages in the presence of antiviral serum, viral membrane antigens are removed from the cell surface and subsequently intracellular viral antigens disappear: Cells look then like uninfected ones by immunofluorescence. In measles SSPE virus-infected C6 rat glioma cells the disappearance of viral antigens is accompanied by full restoration of impaired receptor functions (Barett and Koschel 1983). But the cells are not cured. After removal of viral antiserum viral antigens and the impairments of the receptor system reappear. In the "down modulated" state rabies virus primed cytotoxic T-lymphocytes from C3H mouse do not attack the C3H histocompatibility antigen-bearing rabies virus infected 108CC15 cells. This is shown in Fig. 2A by ^{51}Cr release of the prelabeled target cells. Reappearance of viral antigens after removal of antiviral serum permit an increasing killing of the cells by cytotoxic T-lymphocytes (Fig. 2B).

These observations seem to reflect the situation of persistent virus infections in the CNS where oligclonal antiviral antibodies are present. The results can explain the establishment and maintenance of persistent infections and the fact that persistently infected cells can be controlled by antibodies so that they do not show dysfunctions for a long time. Breakthrough of this immunological control could be the reason for a fast development of virus induced cell destruction enhanced then by immune responses.

Acknowledgment. This work was supported by Sonderforschungsbereich 105 (Project C3) of the DFG.

References

Barret PN, Koschel K (1983) Virology 127:294–308
Fujinami RS, Oldstone MBA (1980) J Immunol 125:78–85
Halbach M, Koschel K (1979) In: Karcher D, Lowenthal A, Strosberg AD (eds) Humoral immunity in neurological diseases. Plenum, New York, pp 499–505
Hamprecht B (1977) Int Rev Cytol 49:99–170
Koschel K, Halbach M (1979) J Gen Virol 42:627–632
Koschel K, Münzel P (1984) Proc Natl Acad Sci USA 81:950–954
Münzel P, Koschel K (1981) Biochem Biophys Res Commun 101:1241–1250

Plasminogen Activator (PA) in Muscle, Its Activation Post-Denervation

B.W. FESTOFF, D. HANTAÏ, C. SORIA, J. SORIA, and M. FARDEAU[1]

1. Introduction

Following injury skeletal muscle undergoes a form of tissue remodelling that can result in relatively complete regeneration (Allbrook 1981). Although the molecular mechanisms underlying this remodelling are not yet understood, the cellular basis resides in the muscle tissue itself. Mammalian skeletal muscle regenerates from activation of quiescent "satellite" cells interposed between plasma and basement membrane (BM) of the muscle fiber. After denervation of mammalian muscle a number of changes also occur. Early events include loss of end-plate specific A_{12} (16 S) acetylcholinesterase (AChE), reduction in fibronectin (Fn) and, invasion of the end-plate by Schwann cells, all within 1–3 days, before muscle atrophy occurs. The possible release of neutral proteases early in denervation may account for the reduction and release of A_{12} AChE (Fernandez et al. 1979), internalization and partial degradation of AChR (Hatzfeld et al. 1982; Romstedt et al. 1983) and of sarcolemmal Fn (Festoff et al. 1977). These changes may be necessary for the re-innervation of denervated muscle fibers, a specialized form of remodelling in this system. Regeneration following muscle freegrafting has been shown to involve changes of Fn, collagen type IV and laminin (Gulati et al. 1983). Remodelling in other systems has been associated with increased activity of serine proteases such as plasminogen activator (PA; Danø et al. 1985), so we were interested in studying PA in skeletal muscle following denervation. Our present results indicate that low levels of PA are present in adult, innervated mouse muscle but that denervation results in a marked time-dependent increase in uPA with modest elevations of tPA. The mol. wt. of the uPA is 48 kd and tPA, 72 kd, consistent with these enzymes studied in other tissues of the mouse (Danø et al. 1985). In addition, potentiators of uPA were found in denervated muscle, and inhibitors for tPA in control muscle.

1   University of Kansas/V.A. Medical Center, Kansas City, MO, USA, and
    Hôpital Lariboisière, Hôtel Dieu and INSERM U 153, Paris, France

Molecular Aspects of Neurobiology
(ed. by Rita Levi Montalcini et al.)
© Springer-Verlag Berlin Heidelberg 1986

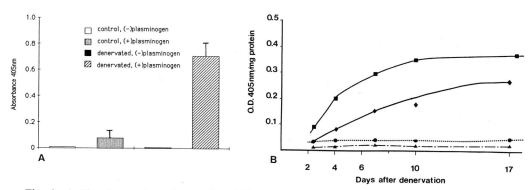

Fig. 1. A Plasminogen-dependence of amidolytic activity of control and denervated muscle extracts. **B** Effect of time of denervation on plasminogen activator of muscle in presence (*square*) or absence (*diamond*) of fibrin monomer

2. Results and Discussion

2.1 Amidolytic Activity

We used an amidolytic assay with a synthetic peptidyl chromogenic substrate (S-2251; KABI, Sweden) specific for plasmin (Ranby et al. 1982) and the activity under our assay conditions was entirely dependent on highly purified human plasminogen (Fig. 1A). This was true for control muscle but strikingly so in the denervated muscle samples. In the current series of experiments, addition of fibrin monomer (Ranby et al. 1982) was used to distinguish uPA from tPA activity in muscle extracts.

2.2 Effects of Denervation on Muscle Plasminogen-dependent Amidolytic Activity

The effect of mid-sciatic neurectomy on muscle PA after different times is shown in Fig. 1B. Only amidolytic activity that was dependent on plasminogen is shown. Plus fibrin PA (upper) increases 8-fold by 7 days post-neurectomy and then plateaus. Without fibrin PA (next lower) rises more gradually but also plateaus. Little or no change in contralateral unoperated muscle PA occurred either in the absence or presence of fibrin monomer (lower curves).

2.3 Fibrin Zymography of Muscle Extracts

We utilized fibrin zymography (Granelli-Piperno and Reich 1978) to confirm the type of PA in muscle. Figure 2 shows a typical fibrin zymogram of control and denervated (different times) muscle extracts. Clear lysis zones at approximately 48 kd were seen with extracts from all denervation times whereas no lysis zones were found with control extracts. The major band of fibrinolytic activity (48 kd) migrates between the high molecular weight (55 kd) uPA and 33 kd uPA. A smaller band, only in late denervation extracts, at 72 kd, co-migrates with pure tPA.

Mr (Kd)

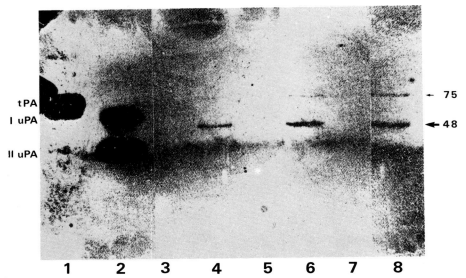

Fig. 2. Fibrin zymography of muscle extracts. *1* Purified human tPA; *2* purified human uPA (55 kd and 33 kd); *3–8* muscle extract for control (*3,5,7*) and denervated (*4,6,8*) for 7 (*3,4*), 10 (*5,6*) and 17 (*7,8*) days. Molecular weight (Mr) in kilodaltons (kd)

2.4 Inhibitors and Potentiators of uPA and tPA in Muscle

To determine if loss of inhibition could account for the marked rise in PA activity in denervated muscle we performed several experiments. To varying amounts of uPA we added buffer, control or denervated extracts without fibrin monomer and measured activity. Surprisingly, the denervated extract significantly potentiated uPA activity with little difference compared to buffer of the control extract (Fig. 3A). We interpreted this to indicate the presence of a potentiator(s) in denervated but no excess, uncomplexed uPA inhibitor in control muscle. On the other hand, incubating varying concentrations of tPA, with control and denervated extracts, in the presence of fibrin monomer resulted in significant inhibition with the control extract. Potentiation, was also found with the denervated extract (Fig. 3B), but the slope of the line was identical to that in buffer only.

3. Summary and Conclusions

We have shown that amidolytic activity for S-2251 in muscle requires plasminogen (Fig. 1A). This PA activity is quite low, perhaps for slow turn-over of extracellular matrix components (see Hantaï and Festoff, this volume). Following denervation, a marked 7-fold rise in PA occurs seen mostly in the absence of added fibrin monomer (Fig. 1B). We interpret this to mean that uPA, not requiring the binding to fibrin (Ranby

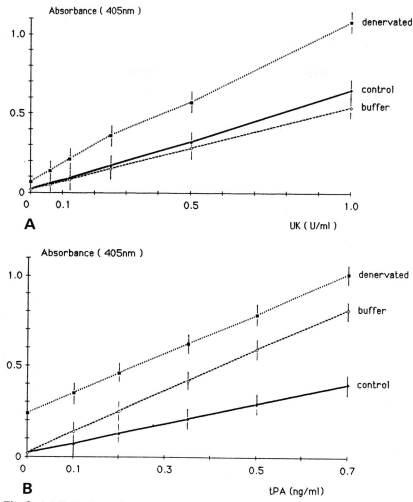

Fig. 3. A Effect of muscle extracts on uPA activity without addition of fibrin monomer. B Effect of muscle extracts on tPA activity in presence of fibrin monomer

et al. 1982; Danø et al. 1985) that characterizes tPA, is predominantly activated. We confirmed this in the fibrin zymogram where we found 48 kd band lysis more intense and occurring sooner after denervation than 72 kd lysis. These molecular weights fit well with those found for mouse uPA and tPA from other tissues (Danø et al. 1985).

We also conclude that some type of potentiator(s) for PA appear in denervated muscle. If this is fibrin or fibrin degradation products then the increased activity (Fig. 3A) may result from a pre-activation of tPA in vivo or at least in situ. It is unlikely the result of in situ plasmin generation since amidolytic activity was completely dependent on exogenous plasminogen (Fig. 1A). Inhibitor(s) also exist for PA in muscle (Fig. 3B). A cellular inhibitor, such as protease nexin already detected in cultured mouse muscle cells (Eaton and Baker 1984), which produce significant PA activity (Festoff et al. 1982), may be responsible. The participation of the PA-plasmin system, as well as other components of fibrinolysis, in the degradation of extracellular BM molecules in denervation and regeneration of skeletal muscle is supported by these results.

Acknowledgments. The authors thank Dr. Olivier Bertrand for purified human plasminogen, Mme A. Thomaidis for help with fibrin zymography, Mlles Sylvie Le Bihan and Pascale Guillaumin for preparation of the manuscript. Performed under a senior research scholarship of the Fulbright Commission in France (to BWF) and a fellowship from the Association des Myopathes de France (to DH). Supported in part by I.N.S.E.R.M., C.N.R.S., NIH (IOINS 17197), ALSSOA and the Medical Research Service of the Veterans Administration.

References

Allbrook D (1981) Skeletal muscle regeneration. Muscle and nerve 4:234−245

Danø K, Andreasen PA, Grøndahl-Hansen J, Kristensen P, Nielsen LS, Skriver L (1985) Plasminogen activators, tissue degradation and cancer. Adv Cancer Res 44:139−266

Eaton DL, Baker JB (1984) Evidence that a variety of cultured cells secrete protease nexin and produce a distinct cytoplasmic serine protease-binding factor. J Cell Physiol 117:175−182

Fernandez HL, Duell MJ, Festoff BW (1979) Neurotrophic regulation of 16 S acetylcholinesterase at the vertebrate neuromuscular junction. J Neurobiol 10:442−454

Festoff BW, Oliver KL, Reddi AB (1977) In vitro studies of skeletal muscle membranes. Effects of denervation on macromolecular components of cation transport in red and white muscle. J Membr Biol 32:345−360

Festoff BW, Patterson MR, Romstedt K (1982) Plasminogen activator: the major secreted neutral protease of cultured skeletal muscle cells. J Cell Physiol 110:190−195

Granelli-Piperno A, Reich E (1978) A study of protease and protease-inhibitor complexes in biological fluids. J Exp Med 148:223−234

Gulati AK, Reddi AH, Zalewski AA (1983) Changes in the basement membrane zone components during skeletal muscle fiber degeneration and regeneration. J Cell Biol 97:957−962

Hatzfeld J, Miskin R, Reich E (1982) Acetylcholine receptor: effects of proteolysis on receptor metabolism. J Cell Biol 92:176−182

Ranby M, Norman B, Wallen P (1982) A sensitive assay for tissue plasminogen activator. Throm Res 27:743−748

Romstedt K, Beach RL, Festoff BW (1983) Studies of acetylcholine receptor turn-over in clonal muscle cells: role of plasmin and effects of protease inhibitors. Muscle and nerve 6:283−290

Adhesive Basement Membrane (BM) Proteins are Degraded by Plasminogen Activator in the Presence of Plasminogen

D. HANTAÏ[1] and B.W. FESTOFF[2]

1. Introduction

The muscle fiber basement membrane (BM) provides tensile strength, ion sieving and scaffolding for regeneration after injury. It serves to keep muscle "satellite" cells interposed between BM and plasma membrane of mammalian muscle fibers. After injury and denervation muscle fibers degenerate or atrophy with activation of stem cells leading to regeneration. Bischoff (1979) showed that in vitro regeneration of single muscle fibers depended on application of neutral proteases to digest the BM. Although recent studies in the frog by McMahan and colleagues (see Sanes 1983) suggest the BM and its components are immutable, other studies in mammals (Gulati et al. 1983) show turn-over of molecules such as fibronectin (Fn; Hynes and Yamada 1982) type IV collagen (coll IV; Timpl et al. 1979a) and laminin (lam; Timpl et al. 1979b). The present study shows that plasmin, generated exogenously or by denervation, degrades BM components with the sensitivity Fn > coll IV > lam. This suggests early participation of the PA-plasmin system in degradation of specific BM components in denervated muscle, in accord with this system's involvement in tissue remodeling occurring in other situations (see Danø et al. 1985).

2. Results and Discussion

2.1 Effect of Various Proteases on BM Antigens

Trypsin applied to 8 μm cryostat sections of mouse sternomastoid muscle caused complete degradation of all BM antigens. No change in relative immunofluorescence (IF; Hantaï et al. 1983) was detected with purified human plasminogen incubated alone for 2 h. Similarly, purified human urokinase (UK55Kd and UK33Kd) had no effect on muscle BM antigens (Fig. 1). When UK55 or UK33 were incubated in the presence of plasminogen, dramatic alterations in IF were found. In Fig. 1D, Fn is

1 INSERM U 153, Paris, France
2 University of Kansas/V.A. Medical Center, Kansas City, MO, USA

Molecular Aspects of Neurobiology
(ed. by Rita Levi Montalcini et al.)
© Springer-Verlag Berlin Heidelberg 1986

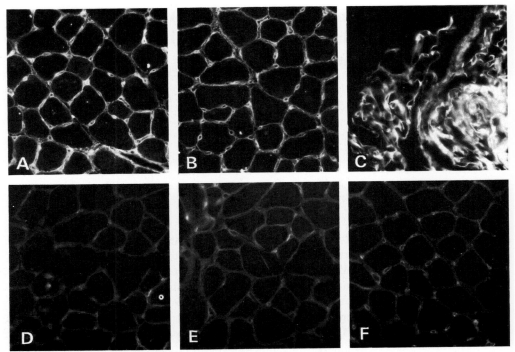

Fig. 1A–F. Plasminogen-dependent exogenous degradation of BM antigens. Fn, control (**A**) and after incubation with UK55Kd (**D**) or control muscle extract (**B**) in presence of plasminogen. Denervated muscle extract and Fn (**E**), lam (**C**) and coll IV (**F**) also in presence of plasminogen. ×100

dramatically reduced in as little as 30 min at 37°C. Reproducibly we found change in appearance of the Fn pattern which was globally decreased. For anti-coll IV the pattern was different. Overall reduction in IF was found with zones of markedly diminished staining giving fibers a "moth-eaten" appearance (Fig. 1F). Interesting results were obtained with anti-sera to lam. The architecture of the fibers remained relatively intact suggesting that neither PA nor plasmin, under these assay conditions, significantly degrades intra-sarcoplasmic proteins. However, reproducibly whole sheets of the extracellular matrix (ECM) sloughed off giving the appearance of a collapsed tent or "geodesic dome" (Fig. 1C). The relative intensity of the collapsed ECM staining for lam was not different from controls. The degradation of an attachment point of lam to the fibers or to some other ECM protein mediating attachment was implied by these results.

2.2 Plasminogen Dependence of BM Degradation by Denervated Muscle Extract

When a 100,000 × g supernatant of normal mouse skeletal muscle homogenates was applied to sections and then antisera applied no observable effects were recorded (Fig. 1B) in the absence or presence of plasminogen. However, when muscle denervated for 10 days was the source of the extract dramatic reduction in IF was seen,

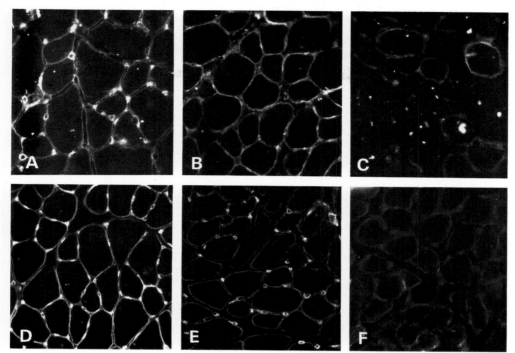

Fig. 2A–F. Denervation-induced degradation of BM antigens. Fn (A–C) and coll IV (D–F) immunofluorescence after incubation with plasminogen for 1 h. Denervation for 2 (A,D), 4 (B,E) and 11 (C,F) days. ×100

similar to effects with purified UK, but again only in the presence of plasminogen (Fig. 1D).

2.3 Qualitative Plasminogen-dependent Degradation After In Vivo Denervation

We studied whether denervation would result in BM antigen changes similar to those found with the free muscle graft model (Gulati et al. 1983). For this, the nerve to the sternomastoid was cut and then muscles removed at 2, 4, 7, 11 and 13 days thereafter. We incubated sections in the absence and presence of plasminogen for the 3 BM antigens. In Fig. 2 the reduction of IF for Fn and coll IV is readily seen during the time course of denervation. No reduction in fluorescent intensity (FI) was found with anti-lam antisera.

2.4 Image Analysis of BM Changes During Muscle Denervation

We next attempted to determine the extent of BM degradation during the time course of denervation. For these studies we utilized a 3 μ diameter, 20 mW laser and a computer program (Albe et al. 1982) to quantitate ECM (endomysial) FI for each antigen.

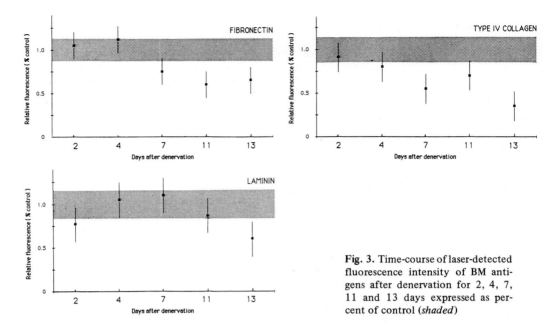

Fig. 3. Time-course of laser-detected fluorescence intensity of BM antigens after denervation for 2, 4, 7, 11 and 13 days expressed as percent of control (*shaded*)

Twenty different fibers were analyzed at each time after denervation (480 total). The results, expressed as percent of control, are shown in Fig. 3. The Fisher test was used to determine significance. For Fn, FI slight decrease at 2 days, then progressive reduction was seen. The extent of reduction compared to the grouped mean of the control is 40% at the level F = 8 ($p < 0.001$). For coll IV reduction begins at day 4 and continues at day 13 to 35% of the control (F = 9, $p < 0.001$). With lam although a trend in FI reduction was seen, it was not significant.

2.5 Summary and Discussion

These studies represent a first attempt to correlate alterations of BM antigens of degenerating skeletal muscle in mammals with PA enzymes capable of degrading these molecules. Elsewhere we have shown that a marked rise in uPA occurs in denervated muscle (Festoff et al., this volume). These results indicate Fn and coll IV are substrates for the plasmin the PAs generate. The question as to which cell of origin of the PAs in muscle is not clear. Clonal mouse muscle cells secrete significant PA (Festoff et al. 1982) but macrophages and other migratory cells may contribute to activated "satellite" cell production. Secondly, what regulates the activation of PA in muscle? Might the nerve regulate muscle PA synthesis or produce one or more PA inhibitors such as protease nexin (Baker et al. 1980). These and other questions will require further studies. The current results implicate the fibrinolytic system in removal of old BM components during muscle injury paving the way for orderly regeneration of the muscle fiber.

Acknowledgments. The authors thank Dr. M. Fardeau for encouragement, Dr. X. Albe for assistance with image analysis. Dr. Olivier Bertrand for the gift of purified human plasminogen, Drs. J. and C. Soria for fruitful discussions and Mlles S. Le Bihan and P. Guillaumin for preparation of the manuscript. Performed under a senior research scholarship of the Fulbright Commission in France (BWF) and a fellowship of the Association des Myopathes de France (DH). Supported in part by I.N.S.E.R.M., NIH (IROINS 17197), ALSSOA and the Medical Research Service of the Veterans Administration.

References

Albe X, Deugnier MA, Caron M, Bisconte JC (1982) A computer-controlled microfluorometer with laser illumination: study of lectin interaction with surfaces of human erythrocytes. Comput Biomed Res 15:563–575

Baker JB, Low DA, Simmer RL, Cunningham DD (1980) Protease nexin: a cellular component that links thrombin and plasminogen activator and mediates their binding to cells. Cell 21:37–45

Bischoff R (1979) Tissue culture studies on the origin of myogenic cells during muscle regeneration in the rat. In: Mauro A (ed) Muscle regeneration. Raven, New York, p 13

Danø K, Andreasen PA, Grøndahl-Hansen J, Kristensen P, Nielsen LS, Skriver L (1985) Plasminogen activators, tissue degradation and cancer. Adv Cancer Res 44:139–266

Festoff BW, Patterson MR, Romstedt K (1982) Plasminogen activator: the major secreted neutral protease of cultured skeletal muscle cells. J Cell Physiol 110:190–195

Gulati AK, Reddi AH, Zalewski AA (1983) Changes in the basement membrane zone components during skeletal muscle fiber degeneration and regeneration. J Cell Biol 97:957–962

Hantaï D, Gautron J, Labat-Robert J (1983) Immunolocalization of fibronectin and other macromolecules of the intercellular matrix in the striated muscle fiber of the adult rat. Collagen Rel Res 3:381–391

Hynes RO, Yamada KM (1982) Fibronectins: multifunctional modular glycoproteins. J Cell Biol 95:369–377

Sanes JR (1983) Roles of extracellular matrix in neural development. Annu Rev Physiol 45:581–600

Timpl R, Rohde H, Gehron Robey P, Rennard SI, Foidart JM, Martin GR (1979a) Laminin: a glycoprotein from basement membranes. J Biol Chem 254:9933–9937

Timpl R, Glanville RW, Wick G, Martin GR (1979b) Immunochemical study on basement membrane (type IV) collagens. Immunology 38:109–116

Soybean Lectin Binding to the Olfactory System of *Xenopus*

B. KEY and P.P. GIORGI[1]

1. Introduction

It is now accepted that cell surface glycans linked to proteins (glycoproteins) or lipids (glycolipids) mediate cell-cell interactions during neurogenesis (Gombos et al. 1978; Edelman 1983). Three main experimental approaches have been used to investigate this aspect of brain development: biochemical analysis of brain homogenates to characterise relevant molecules (Rostas et al. 1979), use of antibodies in cell and tissue cultures (Gallo et al. 1985) and histochemical probing of the brain with antibodies (De Blas et al. 1984) and lectins (Nicolson 1974).

Our laboratory has recently started a systematic investigation of lectin binding to the brain of *Xenopus,* an increasingly popular experimental model for vertebrate brain development. We describe here a very specific binding of soybean agglutinin to the surface of neurons of the olfactory system of *Xenopus borealis,* its developmental pattern and the implications of these findings.

2. Materials and Methods

Concanavalin-A (ConA), soybean agglutinin (SBA), wheat germ agglutinin (WGA) and peanut agglutinin (PNA) were purchased as conjugates to horseradish peroxidase (HRP) from the Sigma Chemical Company.

Larval and young post-metamorphic *Xenopus borealis* were either immersed or perfused fixed with 4% paraformaldehyde. Frozen horizontal sections (40 μm) of the whole animal were cut and processed for lectin binding (Murata et al. 1983).

For electron microscopy 100 μm vibratome sections of the olfactory nerve were incubated and reacted as above.

---

1 Neuroembryology Laboratory, Department of Anatomy, University of Queensland, Brisbane and St. Lucia 4067, Australia

Molecular Aspects of Neurobiology
(ed. by Rita Levi Montalcini et al.)
© Springer-Verlag Berlin Heidelberg 1986

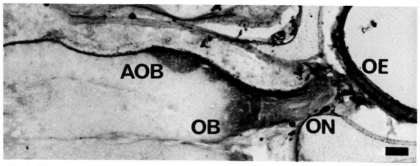

Fig. 1. Horizontal section of *Xenopus* brain (half forebrain represented). SBA-HRP labeling of the olfactory epithelium (*OE*), nerve (*ON*) and bulb (*OB*) and the accessory olfactory bulb (*AOB*). Bar = 250 μm

3. Results

After screening the binding of PNA, ConA, WGA and SBA to the brain of postmeta-morphic *Xenopus* froglets, only SBA revealed a very selective binding pattern, which was restricted to the olfactory system (Fig. 1). The olfactory and vomernasal epithelia, the olfactory and accessory olfactory nerves and the olfactory and accessory olfactory bulbs were all heavily stained, while the rest of the brain (as well as the spinal cord) were free of reaction product. In fact all other regions of the CNS had the same appearance as those in control sections.

In the olfactory epithelium the "olfactory vesicles" (club-like terminal protuber-ances of the distal processes of the olfactory neurons) stood out prominently. The olfactory nerve was intensely labeled by the HRP reaction product throughout its length. The rostral region of the olfactory bulb, containing the olfactory glomeruli (Scalia 1976), the vomeronasal nerve and the accessory olfactory bulb were also intensively labeled (Fig. 1).

The subcellular localization of SBA binding sites in the olfactory nerve was ana-lysed by electron microscopy. Clear accumulation of electron-dense oxidized diamino-benzidine was found around all axons (Fig. 2). Unlike other peripheral nerves, these unmyelinated axons are not individually surrounded by Schwann cell processes, leav-ing no doubt with regard to the cellular localization of binding sites.

A systematic analysis of the *Xenopus* brain from complete sets of serial sections, revealed a further aspect of the SBA binding pattern. A small discrete set of axons on the ventromedial aspect of the forebrain were labeled. These axons appear to arise from the olfactory bulb, some cross to the contralateral side through the anterior commissure while others continue ipsilaterally and cannot be found more caudally than the thalamus. Experimental studies are underway to determine the origin and projections of these axons.

We have investigated the developmental aspects of SBA binding in *Xenopus* brain, and have found that labeling of the olfactory system, as described above, was already present at stage 51 (Niewkoop and Faber 1956).

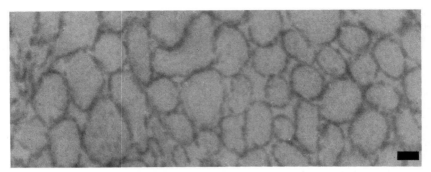

Fig. 2. Electron micrograph of olfactory axons demonstrating surface binding sites for SBA-HRP. The section was not stained with uranyl acetate or lead citrate. Bar = 0.1 μm

4. Discussion

The general aim of probing brain tissue with lectins is to investigate the chemical nature of cell surfaces. The labeling pattern of a lectin becomes experimentally useful when it meets at least two requirements: specificity for a given region or cell type and localization on the cell surface. Both of these requirements are met by SBA binding to *Xenopus* brain. In fact the degree of specificity demonstrated in this case is quite exceptional. To our knowledge this is the first time that a lectin is described to have binding sites only on one cell type in the whole brain. On the other hand, cell surface proteins specific for a given cell type have previously been reported (De Blas et al. 1984).

The fact that one cell type displays a unique characteristic in cell surface composition raises the question of a possible role of SBA-binding sites in recognition and synaptogenesis during development. The appearance of the specific labeling described in this paper at an early developmental stage would suggest such a role, but we do not know as yet if synaptic connections between olfactory axons and their post-synaptic elements are actually formed at that stage in the olfactory pathway. Moreover, labeling by SBA-HRP is not transient, as in the case of ConA and parallel fibres in the cerebellum (Gombos et al. 1978). The persistence of SBA binding sites in post-metamorphic life would suggest a functional, rather than a developmental, role of these surface glycoconjugates. On the other hand, one should keep in mind that the olfactory epithelium of all vertebrates has considerable regenerative capacities. It is possible that cell surface characteristics required during development to establish (or stabilize) connections may be preserved during adult life to subserve regenerative processes. Such a phenomena may explain the maintenance of high concentrations of neural cell adhesion molecule (a cell surface sialoglycoprotein) in the olfactory bulb of adult chick brain (Chuong and Edelman 1983).

Unlike other specific lectin binding reported previously (Gombos et al. 1978), in this case it is possible to dissect a discrete small region of the brain (olfactory bulb) and to characterize SBA-binding sites by affinity chromatography.

Acknowledgments. The authors thank Mrs. P. Bretherton for typing this manuscript. This work was supported by an N.H. & M.R.C. Biomedical Scholarship to B.K. and by an A.R.G.S. grant to P.P.G.

References

Chuong C-M, Edelman GM (1983) Alterations in neural cell adhesion molecules during development of different regions of the nervous system. J Neurosci 4:2354–2368

DeBlas AL, Kuljis RO, Cherwinski HM (1984) Mammalian brain antigens defined by monoconal antibodies. Brain Res 322:277–287

Edelman GM (1983) Cell adhesion molecules. Science 219:450–457

Gallo V, Balazs R, Jorgensen OS (1985) Cell surface proteins of cerebellar interneurones and astrocytes cultured in chemically defined and serum-supplemented media. Dev Brain Res 17:27–37

Gombos G, Vincendon G, Reeber A, Ghandour MS, Zanetta J-P (1978) Membrane glycoproteins in synaptogenesis. In: Neuhoff V (ed) Proceedings of the European Society for Neurochemistry, vol I. Verlag Chemie, New York, p 174

Murata F, Tsuyama S, Suzuki S, Hamada H, Ozawa M, Muramatsu T (1983) Distribution of glycoconjugates in the kidney studied by use of labelled lectins. J Histochem Cytochem 31:139–144

Nicolson GL (1974) The interactions of lectins with animal cell surface. Int Rev Cytol 39:89–190

Nieuwkoop PD, Faber J (1956) Normal table of *Xenopus laevis* (Daudin). North Holland, Amsterdam

Rostas JAP, Kelly PT, Pesin RH, Cotman CW (1979) Protein and glycoprotein composition of synaptic junctions prepared from discrete synaptic regions and different species. Brain Res 168:151–167

Scalia F (1976) Structure of the olfactory and accessory olfactory systems. In: Llinas R, Precht W (eds) Frog neurobiology. Springer, Berlin Heidelberg New York, p 213

Isolation of cDNA Clones Encoding Neurofilament Proteins

J.-P. JULIEN, D. MEYER, W. MUSHYNSKI, and F. GROSVELD[1]

1. Introduction

Each type of intermediate filament (IF) is composed of biochemically distinct proteins which are differentially expressed in different tissues: cytokeratin filaments are found in epithelial cells, vimentin in cells of mesenchymal origin, desmin in muscle cells, glial filaments in glial cells and neurofilaments (NFs) in neurons (Lazarides 1980). IF genes appear to be derived from a common ancestral gene, e.g. comparison between keratin and vimentin genes has shown that the intron positions are highly conserved, in spite of substantial sequence divergence between these IF genes (Lehnert et al. 1984; Marchuk et al. 1984).

The three NF proteins with apparent molecular weights of 68K (NF68), 145K (NF145) and 200K (NF200) on SDS-gel electrophoresis share with other types of IF proteins a homologous α-helical domain, but contain long extensions at their carboxy terminals responsible for their differences in size (Julien and Mushynski 1983; Geisler et al. 1983). We report here the isolation of cDNA clones encoding the murine NF68 and NF145 proteins.

2. Results and Discussion

Synthetic oligonucleotide probes complementary to the mRNA of peptides located in the α-helix and the carboxy terminal regions of NF68 protein have been used to isolate a cDNA clone from the rat (Julien et al. 1985). The 900bp insert cloned in pBr322 spans the helix 1b and helix II as well as part of the carboxy terminal domain of NF68 protein (data not shown).

To obtain a larger NF68 cDNA we have subsequently prepared a library in bacteriophage λgt10 from polyA$^+$ RNA of mouse brain. Screening of 5×10^5 recom-

1 Laboratory of Gene Structure and Expression, National Institute for Medical Research, The Ridgeway, Mill Hill, London NW7 1AA, Great Britain

Molecular Aspects of Neurobiology
(ed. by Rita Levi Montalcini et al.)
© Springer-Verlag Berlin Heidelberg 1986

binants with the rat NF68 probe yielded 46 positively hybridizing plaques. The largest insert of 2.6 kb was subcloned into the plasmid vector pUC8 for analysis.

Partial nucleotide sequence of this mouse NF68 cDNA is shown in Fig. 1. It spans the entire coding region of the mouse NF68 gene, 541 residues corresponding to a molecular mass of 61K. There is a polyadenylation site AATAAA at 290 nucleotides downstream from the translational stop codon TGA. Preliminary S1 nuclease mapping experiments indicate that this cDNA clone contains 30 nucleotides upstream of the ATG initiating codon.

A comparison of the mouse with the rat (Julien et al. 1985) and porcine sequences (Geisler et al. 1985) indicates a high degree of conservation of NF68 protein. However, the divergence is not evenly spread over the different domains of NF68 protein. Between the mouse and the pig there is only 4% and 2% divergence in the amino terminal and helical regions, respectively, whereas a substantial divergence (>20%) occurs in the highly charged tail regions. This appears to be the result of a number of duplication/deletion events of a core DNA sequence coding for charged amino acid residues. The high degree of divergence indicates that the charge, rather than the primary sequence and/or secondary structure of the tail is important.

Southern blot analysis suggests that the NF68 gene is a single copy gene (Julien et al. 1985; Lewis and Cowan 1985). However, Northern blot hybridization reveals the presence of two poly A^+ mRNA species of 3.4 and 2.4 kb (Fig. 2A). At present we do not know whether both RNA species are translated into a functionally active protein. It is unlikely that these equally abundant transcripts are derived from alternative polyadenylation sites at the 3' end of the NF gene. Work is in progress shows that the multiple transcripts are not generated from different initiation sites of transcription or from alternative splicing of the same RNA precursor. Northern blot analysis (Fig. 2B) shows that NF68 mRNAs are co-expressed during brain development. Both species are detected in the 11d embryonic brain. There is a slight increase in the mRNA levels during embryonic development until birth, which is followed by a large increase in the postnatal brain, coinciding with the time of axonal elongation.

3. Cloning of an NF145 cDNA

The isolation of NF145 cDNA clones was based on cross-hybridization with the NF68 cDNA probe, since it was known that the NF68 and NF145 proteins share significant homologies in sequence (Geisler et al. 1985). In addition, hybrid selection experiments carried out at reduced stringency indicated that an NF68 cDNA probe was able to detect mRNA encoding the NF145 protein (Lewis and Cowan 1985). As expected, screening of our cDNA library with an NF68 probe at reduced stringency yielded several cross-hybridizing clones, two of which were found to encode NF145 protein. The partial sequence of an NF145 cDNA clone of 900bp in size is shown in Fig. 3. The deduced protein sequence is identical to the corresponding por-

```
                    S   S   F   G   Y   D   P   Y   F   S   T   S   Y   K   R   Y   V   E   T   P   R   V
ACCACTGGTCTCCTGCCCCACTGCAGTCACC ATG AGT TCG TTC GGC TAC GAT CCG TAC TTT TCG ACC TCC TAC AAG CGG TAT GTG GAG ACG CCC CGG GTG

24   H   I   S   V   R   S   G   Y   S   T   A   R   S   A   Y   S   S   V   R   S
     CAC ATC TCC GTG CGC AGC GGC TAC AGC ACG GCG CGC TCC GCC TAC TCG TCC GTC CGC AGC

56   Y   S   S   S   G   S   L   M   P   S   L   E   N   L   D   L   S   Q   V   A   I   S   N   D   L   K   S   I   R   T
     TAC TCC AGC TCT GGC TCT TTG ATG CCC AGC CTG GAG AAT CTC GAT CTG AGC CAG GTA GCC ATC AGC AAC GAC CTC AAG TCT ATC CGC ACA

88   Q   E   K   A   Q   L   Q   D   L   N   D   R   F   A   S   F   I   E   R   V   H   E   L   E   Q   N   K   V   L   E   A
     CAA GAG AAG GCA CAG CTG CAG GAC CTC AAC GAT CGC TTC GCC AGC TTC ATC GAG CGC GTC CAT GAG CTG GAG CAG AAC AAG GTC TTG GAA GCC

120  E   L   L   V   L   K   Q   K   H   S   E   P   S   R   F   R   A   L   Y   E   Q   E   I   R   D   L   R   L   A   A   E   D
     GAG CTG CTG GTG CTG AAA CAG AAA CAC CAC TCT GAG CCT TCC CGC TTC CGC GCC CTG TAC GAG CAG GAG ATC CGC GAT CTG CGC CTG GCA GCG GAA GAC

152  A   T   N   E   K   Q   A   L   Q   G   E   R   E   G   L   E   E   T   L   R   N   L   Q   A   R   Y   E   E   E   V   L
     GCC ACT AAC GAG AAG CAA GCC CTT CAA GGC GAG CGC GAG GGG CTG GAG GAG ACT CTG CGC AAC CTG CAG GCT CGC TAT GAG GAA GTG CTG

184  S   K   E   D   Q   G   R   L   M   E   A   R   K   G   A   D   E   A   L   R   A   E   L   K   R   I   D   S   L   M
     AGC CGC GAG GAC CAG GGC CGG CTG ATG GAA GCG CGC AAA GGC GCG GAT GAG GCC CTC CGC GCC GAG CTG AAG CGC ATC GAC AGC CTG ATG

216  D   E   I   A   F   L   K   K   V   H   E   E   E   I   A   E   L   Q   A   Q   I   Q   Y   A   Q   I   S   V   E   M   D   V
     GAC GAG ATA GCT TTC CTG AAG AAG GTG CAC GAG GAA ATC GCC GAG CTG CAG GCT CAG ATC CAG TAT GCT CAG ATC TCC GTG GAG ATG GAC GTG

248  S   S   K   P   D   L   S   A   A   L   K   D   I   R   A   Q   Y   E   K   L   A   A   K   N   M   Q   N   A   E   E   W   F
     TCC TCC AAG CCC GAC CTC TCC GCC GCT CTC AAG GAC ATC CGC GCT CAG TAC GAG AAG CTG GCC GCC AAG AAC ATG CAG AAC GCC GAA GAG TGG TTC

280  K   S   R   F   T   V   L   T   E   S   A   A   K   N   T   D   A   V   R   A   A   K   D   E   V   S   E   S   R   R   L   L
     AAG AGC CGC TTC ACC GTG CTA ACC GAG AGC GCC GCC AAG AAC ACC GAC GCT GTG CGC GCT GCC AAG GAC GAG GTG TCG GAA AGC CGG CGC CTG CTC
```

```
312
K   A   K   T   L   E   I   E   A   C   R   G   H   N   E   A   L   E   K   Q   L   Q   E   L   E   D   K   Q   N   A   D   I
AAG GCT AAG ACC CTG GAG ATC GAA GCC TGC CGG GGT ATG AAC GAA GCT CTG GAG AAG CAG CTG CAG GAG CTA GAG GAC AAG CAG AAT GCA GAC ATT

344
S   A   M   Q   D   T   I   Q   K   L   E   N   E   L   R   S   T   K   S   E   H   A   R   Y   L   K   E   Y   Q   D   L   L
AGC GCC ATG CAG GAC ACA ATC AAC AAG CTG GAG AAT GAG CTG AGA AGC ACG AAG AGC ATG GCC AGG TAC CTG AAG GAG TAC CAG GAC CTC CTC

376
N   V   K   M   A   L   D   I   E   I   A   A   Y   R   K   L   L   E   G   E   E   T   R   L  S/F  T   S   V   G.  I
AAT GTC AAG ATG GCC TTG GAC ATC GAG ATT GCA GCT TAC AGA AAA CTC TTG GAA GGC GAA GAG ACC AGG CTC AGT TTC ACC AGC GTG GGT AGC ATA

408
T   S   G   Y   S   Q   S   Q   V   F   G   R   S   A   Y   S   G   L   Q   S   S   Y   L   M   S   A   R   S   F   P
ACC AGC GGC TAC TCT CAG AGC TCG CAG GTC TTC GGC CGT TCT GCT TAC AGT GGC TTG CAG AGC TCC TAC TTG ATG TCT GCT CGC TCT TTC CCA

440
A   Y   Y   T   S   H   V   Q   E   E   Q   T   E   V   E   E   T   I   E   A   T   K   A   E   E   A   K   D   E   P   P   S
GCC TAC TAT ACC AGC CAC GTC CAG GAA CAG ACA GAG GTC GAG GAG ACC ATT GAG GCT ACG AAA GCT GAG GAG GCC AAG GAT GAG CCC CCC TCT

472
E   G   E   A   E   E   E   K   E   K   E   G   E   E   E   E   E   A   E   E   D
GAA GGA GAA GCA GAA GAG GAG AAG GAG AAG GAG GGA GAA GAG GAG GAA GCT GCC AAG GAT GAG TCT GAA GAC

504
T   K   E   E   E   G   E   G   E   E   D   T   K   E   S   E   E   E   E   K   K   E   E   S   A   G   E   E   Q
ACA AAA GAA GAA GAA GGT GGT GAG GGT GAG GAG GAG GAC ACC AAA GAA TCT GAA GAG GAA GAG AAG AAG GAA GAG AGT GCT GGA GAG GAG CAG

536
V   A   K   K   K   D
GTG GCT AAG AAG AAG GAT TGA GCCCTATTCCCAACTATTCCAGGAAAAGTCTCCCAATCAGGTCCAACCTCATCACCAACCAGTTGAGTTCGAGATCCTATACAAATTAAGAAG

TCAATACATGTATAATTCTGAGATGACTTAGGTTGGACTTTCAATGTTGTGTCTATGAATTCCTCCTTACGCAGAGTATCTGTTTGCTTGCAGAGTGGCTTTCTGGCTTGCTGCCAGCCTGTGCATG

GTCCATGCTTATGAGTTCAGGATCTATGGCAATGTGAATCACACAGATGTTTACAATAATAATAAAAAAAAAAACCACCACCACAC
```

Fig. 1. Nucleotide sequence of a mouse NF68 cDNA clone. The nucleotide sequence was determined by the methods of Maxam and Gilbert (1980) and by the M13-dideoxy strategy (Sanger et al. 1980). The predicted amino acid sequence of the open reading frame is shown above the DNA sequence. The α-helixal regions typical of IF proteins are *boxed*

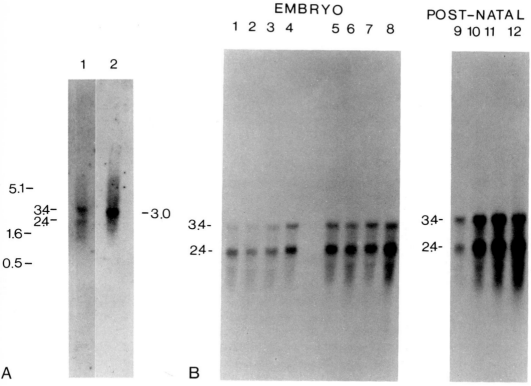

Fig. 2. A RNA blot hybridization of 10 µg of mouse brain RNA with a mouse NF68 cDNA probe (*lane 1*) and NF145 cDNA probe (*lane 2*). The marker sizes were obtained from λ and PBR322 digests (kb). **B** Expression of NF68 during mouse brain development. Each *lane* contains 10 µg of total brain RNA obtained at different stages of development: on the *left panel* (embryo) *lanes 1 to 8* represent respectively 11d, 12d, 13d, 15d, 16d, 17d, 18d and new born brain: on the *right* panel *lanes 9 to 12* represent respectively newborn, 9d, 15d and adult brain

Fig. 3. Partial nucleotide sequence of NF145 cDNA. The nucleotide sequence was determined by the M13-dideoxy strategy. The predicted amino acid sequence is shown above the DNA sequence

```
1
L    Q    S    K    S    I    E    L    E    S    V    R    G    T    K    E
CTG  CAG  TCC  AAG  AGC  ATC  GAG  CTC  GAG  TCG  GTG  CGA  GGC  ATT  AAG  GAG

33
L    S    S    Y    Q    D    T    I    Q    Q    L    E    N    E    L    R
CTC  AGC  AGC  TAC  CAG  GAC  ACC  ATC  CAG  CAG  TTG  GAA  AAT  GAA  CTT  CGG

65
L    N    V    K    M    A    L    D    I    E    I    A    A    Y    R    K
CTT  AAC  GTC  AAG  ATG  GCC  CTG  GAC  ATC  GAG  ATC  GCC  GCG  TAC  AGG  AAA
```

cine NF145 proteins (Geisler et al. 1985). A comparison at the nucleic acid level between NF145 and NF68 reveals a region (residues 60–88) with only 16% divergence. We believe that this region which corresponds to the most highly conserved consensus sequence of IF proteins is responsible for the observed cross-hybridization.

Southern blot analysis suggests the presence of a single NF145 gene (not shown), while the NF145 probe detects a single 3.0kb mRNA on Northern blots (Fig. 2A).

The availability of cDNA probes has recently allowed us to isolate the genomic copies of NF68 and NF145 genes. Sequencing and structural studies of these genes is presently in progress.

References

Geisler N, Kaufmann E, Fisher S, Plessmann U, Weber K (1983) EMBO J 2:1295–1302
Geisler N, Plessmann V, Weber K (1985) FEBS Lett 182:475–479
Julien J-P, Mushynski WE (1983) J Biol Chem 258:4019–1025
Julien J-P, Ramachandran K, Grosveld F (1985) Biochem Biophys Acta (in press)
Lazarides E (1980) Nature 283:249–256
Lehnert ME, Jorcano JL, Zentgrafs H, Blessing M, Franz JK, Franke WW (1984) EMBO J 3: 3279–3287
Lewis SA, Cowan NJ (1985) J Cell Biol 100:843–850
Marchuk D, McCrohon S, Fuchs E (1984) Cell 39:491–498
Maxam A, Gilbert W (1980) Methods in enzymology. Academic, New York, 65:499–560
Sanger F, Coulson AR, Barrel BG, Smith AJH, Roe BA (1980) J Mol Biol 143:161–178

S	L	E	R	Q	L	S	D	I	E	E	R	H	N	H	D
TCC	CTG	GAG	CGG	CAG	CTC	AGC	GAC	ATC	GAG	GAG	CGC	CAC	AAC	CAC	GAC

G	T	K	W	E	M	A	R	H	L	R	E	Y	Q	D	L
GGA	ACC	AAG	TGG	GAA	ATG	GCT	CGT	CAT	TTG	CGA	GAA	TAC	CAG	GAT	CTC

L	L	E	G	E	E	T	R	F	S	T	F
CTC	CTA	GAG	GGG	GAA	GAG	ACC	AGA	TTT	AGC	ACA	TTT

The Murine Thy-1 Gene

V. GIGUERE and F. GROSVELD[1]

1. Introduction

The Thy-1 antigen is a small glycoprotein found in large amounts at the cell surface
of brain cells and rodent thymocytes, and in lesser quantities on a number of other
tissues (Campbell et al. 1981). In many of these tissues, the level of expression of
Thy-1 has been shown to vary during differentiation in the mouse, Thy-1 occurs in
two allotypic forms referred to as Thy-1.1 (AKR) and Thy-1.2 (Balb/c and others)
(Reif and Allen 1964) coded for by a gene that maps on chromosome 9 (Blankenhorn
and Douglas 1972). In contrast, in humans only one allotypic form is known coded
for by a gene that maps on chromosome 11 (van Rijs et al. 1985). Structural and
sequence homologies between the Thy-1 glycoprotein and immunoglobulin (Ig)
domains and other members of the Ig superfamily have led to the suggestion that
Thy-1 may represent the primordial Ig domain (Williams and Gagnon 1982) lending
support to the argument that the immune system may have evolved from the nervous
system. Thus, the study of the Thy-1 gene is interesting, both from the point of view
of its structure and the mechanisms which control its tissue-specific expression.

2. Results and Discussion

We have cloned the genes encoding the two allotypic forms of the mouse Thy-1
antigen and the structure of the mouse Thy-1.2 gene has been determined (Giguere et
al. 1985). The gene consists of four exons, which correspond approximately to the
functional domains of the protein. The transcription unit of the mouse gene span
6 kb of genomic DNA of which the coding and non-coding regions total 1700 bp after
processing (Fig. 1). This is consistent with a size of 1850 nt determined for the Thy-1
mRNA on Northern blots (Giguere et al. 1985), assuming a polyA tail of about 150 nt.
Using primer extension and S1 nuclease mapping assays, we have defined the borders
of the transcriptional unit (Giguere et al. 1985). The Thy-1 mRNA has multiple sites

1   Laboratory of Gene Structure and Expression, National Institute for Medical Research,
    The Ridgeway, Mill Hill, London NW7 1AA, Great Britain

Molecular Aspects of Neurobiology
(ed. by Rita Levi Montalcini et al.)
© Springer-Verlag Berlin Heidelberg 1986

of transcription initiation at the 5' end, and a single polyadenylation site at the 3' end of the gene (Fig. 1).

Although the physiological role of Thy-1 is still not clear, the analysis of its exon/intron structure fully confirms its homology with the Ig superfamily of proteins (Williams and Gagnon 1982), the different functional domains of the protein are encoded on separate exons with the exception of the 5' leader sequence of the gene which is divided over two exons. This property is shared by β2 microglobulin, the only other published protein in the Ig superfamily that contains a single extra cellular domain. Thy-1 might therefore be more closely related to β2-microglobulin than was suggested by Hood et al. (1985). Comparison of the Thy-1 genes from different mouse strains (Giguere et al. 1985) shows that the Thy-1.1 gene is more similar to the C57/B6 Thy-1.2 (Seki et al. 1985) than is the Balb/c Thy-1.2 gene. At present we do not know whether this indicates a high degree of polymorphism of the Thy-1 gene or whether this represent a very limited number of variant genes propagated by inbreeding.

The mouse Thy-1 glycoprotein is expressed in a developmental stage and tissue-specific manner, its highest levels being found at the cell surface of thymocytes and brain cells. Recently, reintroduction of a cloned Thy-1.2 gene into different cell lines showed that the resulting transformants express up to 50-fold more cell surface Thy-1.2 antigen when the cell lines transformed already expressed the Thy-1 antigen at its cell surface (Evans et al. 1984). Although no data on the levels of the Thy-1 mRNA were presented, these results suggest that the Thy-1 gene might be subject to cell-specific transcriptional control. Thus, analysis of the mouse Thy-1 gene structure is a crucial first step towards studying the mechanisms which regulate its expression. Interestingly, the sequence analysis (Fig. 1) reveals that the Thy-1 gene contains an unusual promoter. The immediate 5' flanking of the putative CAP site contains a relatively high G/C content (68%) and lacks the conserved TATA and CAAT boxes found in the majority of eukaryotic promoters. For most of the genes that lack these sequences, the absence of a conserved TATA box produces mRNAs whose 5' termini are heterogeneous, a phenomenon also observed for the Thy-1 mRNA (Fig. 1). In comparison with the genes mentioned above, only one strong region of homology can be detected, i.e. at position −34 in the Thy-1 gene with the corresponding region of the mouse DHFR gene. This makes the Thy-1 promoter rather unique and we have initiated deletion and linker scanning mutant studies to identify sequences responsible for the correct initiation of the Thy-1 mRNA per se (Fig. 2). The Thy-1 5' flanking sequences and first exon with different deletions were linked to the chloramphenicol acetyl transferase (CAT) gene (Gorman et al. 1982). This reporter gene plasmid also contains an SV40 enhancer at its 3' end. The different plasmids were introduced into L-cells by Ca phosphate precipitation and the cells were analyzed 60 h later for CAT activity (Gorman et al. 1982). Figure 2 shows that the removal of sequences between −116 and −86 from the major cap site reduces the activity of the gene to 5% of its original level. Further deletions which remove all of the flanking sequences reduce this remnant activity to a 1% background level. From these preliminary results, we conclude that an upstream element around −100 is responsible for the activity of the Thy-1 promoter. The most obvious candidate sequence for this function is a run of pyrimidine nucleotides in this region (see Fig. 1).

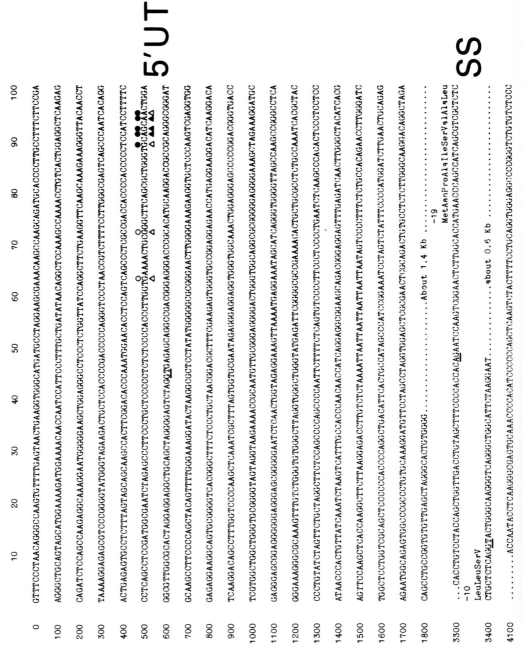

Fig. 1. DNA sequence of the mouse Thy-1.2 gene. The amino acid sequence is shown above the DNA sequence. The splice signal dinucleotides GT and AG and the polyadenylation signal AATAAA are underlined. The location of the mRNA cap sites as determined by S1 nuclease and primer extension analysis are indicated by *circles* and *triangles*, respectively. *Open symbols* indicate

weak bands on the autoradiographs. A second first exon with its own promoter has recently been identified (Ingraham et al. 1986; Spanopoulou, unpubl.), i.e. the gene has two independent promoters with a first exon which splice onto the same second exon. The alternative first exon is located at positions 854–994

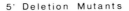

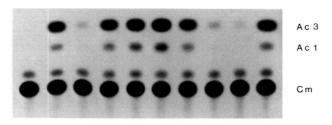

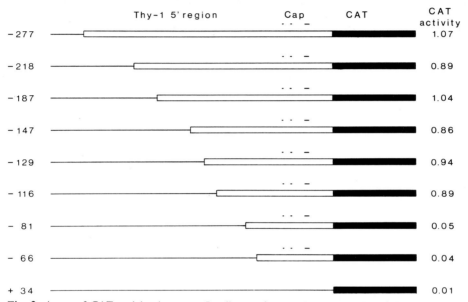

Fig. 2. Assay of CAT activity in mouse L-cells transfected with deletion Thy-1-CAT constructs. Cells were transfected with 10 μg of DNA and assayed 60 h later for CAT activity. The *top panel* shows a CAT assay of the deletion mutants indicated in the *bottom panel*. The activity of each construct was quantitated from several experiments and normalized to the non-deleted plasmid

In addition, preliminary results suggest that more than just the 5′ end of the gene is required to obtain tissue specific expression (Giguere, unpublished).

Previous studies have shown that the Thy-1 antigen can be detected on differentiated embryonal carcinoma cells. This observation is confirmed for EC cells at the level of Thy-1 mRNA (Giguere et al. 1985). At present we cannot distinguish between the two possible mechanisms for the increase of the mRNA; either stabilization of Thy-1 mRNA (which was rapidly turned over before differentiation) or alternatively, a transcriptional activation. Either way, since EC cells can be differentiated to give several different cell types, including neuronal cells, and since they can be transformed by DNA mediated gene transfer and give rise to regulated expression of exogenous genes, this should provide an interesting system to study the early expression of Thy-1.

References

Blankenhorn E, Douglas T (1972) J Hered 63:259–263

Campbell DG, Gagnon J, Reid KBM, Williams AF (1981) Biochem J 195:1–30

Evans GA, Ingraham HA, Lervis K, Cunningham K, Seki T, Moriuchi T, Chang HC, Silver J, Hyman R (1984) Proc Natl Acad Sci USA 81:5532–5534

Giguere V, Isobe K-I, Grosveld FG (1985) EMBO J 4:2017–2024

Gorman C, Moffat L, Howard B (1982) Mol Cell Biol 2:1044–1051

Hood L, Kronenberg M, Hunkapiller T (1985) Cell 40:225–229

Reif A, Allen J (1964) J Exp Med 120:413–433

Seki T, Chang H-C, Meriuchi T, Denome R, Ploegh H, Silver J (1985) Science 227:649–651

van Rijs J, Giguere V, Hurst J, Agthoven T, Goyert S, Grosveld FG (1985) Proc Natl Acad Sci USA 82:5832–5835

Williams AF, Gagnon J (1982) Science 216:696–703

Molecular Diversity and Neuronal Function

F.E. BLOOM[1]

1. Introduction

The patriarch of American neuroscience, Professor F.O. Schmitt (1984) has recently (1984) defined the transitions and conceptual upheavals that new data are forcing. Onto the classical, hard-wired nervous system of our training years has been super-imposed a much looser nervous system in which neurons may release their signals to act, at unknown distances from the release site, not strictly as primary communicators, but rather as signals that can modify the response of the intended target cells to their other afferent signals. In less than one decade, the nervous system ceased to be a rather dry place in which, to classic physiologists, transmitters meant relatively little, since they all worked either to excite or inhibit. In its stead we have a very juicy, flexible nervous system in which transmitters act on many different receptor transduction mechanisms to provide a very enriched repertoire of signalling capabilities across widely differing spatial domains and widely variant durations of action that provide through the analysis of specific molecular mechanisms, a highly enriched diversity of response capacity. For this communication, I will concentrate my remarks on three accumulations of our data that seem relevant to these concerns.

2. Monoaminergic Systems Provide Specific Mechanisms of Diversity

Monoamines were among the first chemically defined transmitters to meet the more rigorous tests as central transmitters. This was due to three specific advantages: the broader armamentarium of drugs available to manipulate the central monoaminergic systems, the detailed structural information on these systems resulting from specific and sensitive methods for their cytochemical localizations and the fact that the major source of noradrenergic axons to easily identified target neurons in cerebellum and cortex were clustered in an easily stimulated pontine nucleus, the locus coeruleus (see Foote et al. 1983). However, their highly divergent axonal projections and their

---

1   Division of Preclinical Neuroscience and Endocrinology, Scripps Clinic and Research Foundation, 10666 North Torrey Pines Road, La Jolla, CA 92037, USA

Molecular Aspects of Neurobiology
(ed. by Rita Levi Montalcini et al.)
© Springer-Verlag Berlin Heidelberg 1986

unique electrophysiological actions — altering membrane potential without increased ionic conductance (see Foote et al. 1983; Siggins and Gruol 1986 for recent reviews) — required considerable conceptual expansion of the concept of a neurotransmitter.

3. Cortical Organization of Noradrenergic Circuits

The continued analysis of the NA coeruleo-cortical system in the rat, has demonstrated two major characteristics: (1) there is a rich network of NA innervation throughout all layers and regions of the dorsal and lateral cortex which is characterized by a relatively uniform laminar pattern, and (2) the major NA fibers are oriented and travel longitudinally through the grey matter and branch widely (see Morrison and Magistretti 1983; Magistretti and Morrison 1985). Thus, the NA innervation of neocortex may be viewed as tangential afferent system whose organization and pattern of termination is different from the highly localized, radial nature of the thalamo-cortical afferents.

More recent studies of monoamines in the far more highly differentiated, gyrencephalic neocortex of the primate brain have shown the need for considerable refinement in concepts of monoamine circuit specificity. We find that the specific density and pattern of NA (or 5-HT) innervation in a particular cortical locus varies systematically as a function of several factors: the cytoarchitectonic region, the cortical lamina, the species of animal, age of the animal, and the functional interaction of the region with other. Each of these factors influences monoaminergic innervation patterns specifically, and have been described in detail in our recent publications (Foote and Morrison 1984). More recently, my colleagues undertook a detailed examination of primate primary visual cortex to evaluate the degree of laminar specialization within the most laminarly specialized region of the neocortex.

These two fiber systems, indeed, exhibited a high degree of laminar specialization, and were, in fact, distributed in a complementary fashion: layers V and VI receive a moderately dense NA projection and a sparse 5-HT projection, whereas layers IVa and IVc receive a very dense 5-HT projection and are largely devoid of NA fibers. These patterns of innervation imply that the two transmitter systems affect different stages of cortical information processing: the raphe-cortical 5-HT projections may preferentially innervate the spiny stellate cells of layers IVa and IVc, whereas the coeruleo-cortical NA projection may be directed predominantly at pyramidal cells.

4. Interactions Between Vasoactive Intestinal Polypeptide and Noradrenaline in Rat Cerebral Cortex

The complementary, non-overlapping innervation of neocortical target areas by NA and 5-HT systems, represents one form of transmitter diversity. A different sort of diversity emerges from comparison of the NA afferents with the intrinsic cortical VIP-containing bipolar neurons. Several lines of evidence support a role for vasoactive intestinal polypeptide (VIP) as a neuronal messenger in cerebral cortex. Biochemical data support its presence, release, binding, and at least one possible action (see Morrison and Magistretti 1983; Magistretti and Morrison 1985, for refs.). Significant actions of VIP on central neurons include the ability to stimulate cyclic AMP formation in cortical slices with greater potency than noradrenaline (NA).

Cytochemically, VIP and NA containing circuits show a contrasting but complementary cortical anatomy (see Morrison and Magistretti 1983): VIP neurons are intrinsic, bipolar, radially oriented, intracortical neurons (Morrison and Magistretti 1983) while the NA system innervates a broad expanse of cortex in a horizontal plane. Yet the two fiber systems may have the same targets, the pyramidal cells. Identified cortical pyramidal neurons are depressed in spontaneous firing by iontophoresis of either NA or cyclic AMP (see Foote et al. 1983). The recent findings of Magistretti and Schorderet (1985) suggest that VIP and NA can act synergistically to increase cyclic AMP in cerebral cortex. Therefore, we tested VIP and NA on rat cortical neurons to evaluate this interaction at the cellular level using iontophoresis. Analysis of more than 100 cortical neurons suggests definitively that there are significant interactions: application of VIP during subthreshold NA administration causes pronounced inhibitions of cellular discharge regardless of the effect of VIP prior to NA (Ferron et al. 1985). Even in cases where VIP alone gave excitatory effects, concurrent subthreshold NA treatment reversed the VIP effect from excitation to inhibition.

Magistretti and Schorderet (1985) also showed that the synergism of VIP by NA was blocked by phentolamine, an alpha adrenergic receptor antaginist, and mimicked by phenylephrine, an alpha receptor agonist. Accordingly, we examined, and observed, that phenylephrine pretreatment give equivalent synergistic effects on VIP actions to those of NA (Ferron et al. 1984). Thus, the interaction of VIP and NA at the cellular level may also involve alpha receptor activation, although further testing is required. If NA and VIP-containing fibers do indeed converge on the same cortical target cell, it is feasible that cyclic AMP is the intracellular mediator of their synergistic interaction.

5. Diversity in Other Systems

Space does not permit here an exploration of the extensive diversity in intercellular chemical signalling that would seem to be available through the temporal and spatial convergence of classical transmitter systems and conditional transmitter systems such as the monoamines and peptides. Elsewhere (see Bloom 1984a,b) I have hypothesized that "conditional" transmitter actions are those in which the magnitude and quality of a given target cell's response to its afferents will be conditional, depending on which of these regulatory afferent systems are simultaneously active.

There would also seem to be quite enough differently acting, differently constituted transmitter systems already available, in the amino acids, the monoamines and the peptides, each with their own intrinsic patterns of circuitry, and a surprising degree of added co-existence. Nevertheless, it must be recognized that the transmitter systems available for analysis now have been largely discovered through trial and error searches

factors (see Bloom 1984a). Recently my colleagues and I (see Sutcliffe et al. 1983, 1984) initiated a more comprehensive search for transmitters and other unique molecules important to the regulation of neuronal activity by exploiting the powerful methods of molecular biology.

Although we have made extensive progress in identifying novel brain proteins, including one potential new family of neuropeptides, the main major insight from those studies for the present discourse is the recognition that more than 60% of the genome may be selectively expressed in brain, amounting to no less than 30,000 "brain-specific" proteins, including — one must conclude — more than just a few new neuropeptides, and other messenger molecules. Therefore, it is clear that the divergence in mechanisms of synaptic diversity is nowhere near a conclusion and that simplifying principles must be found to begin to integrate this complex picture.

6. Conclusions

The study of the central monoaminergic systems, especially the comprehensive anatomy, physiology and behavioral studies that have been compiled for the central noradrenergic neurons has clearly broadened the concept of neurotransmitter actions and synaptic system interactions. There are many, many peptides to be added eventually into this system of interactions, assuming that the rules for documenting them as transmitters, or co-transmitters, will eventually expand beyond the present anatomic evidence of their existence within nerve terminals.

However, there are as yet no comparable physiological synaptic data for peptide-containing systems in which a clustered group of neurons is susceptible to activation and recording under conditions that would define the possible time and space properties of the responses of the likely target cells. In fact, there are not instances of which I am aware in which the effects of a peptide containing system in the mammalian CNS have been shown conclusively to be peptidergic.

While we are not totally ready to set aside all of our historical precedents in transmitter research, it does seem clear that the complexity and abundance of already identified messages in the brain demands that we keep an open mind about the kinds of factors and their functions that may be found if we are not to be doomed to saying that all we know now is all there can ever be. The interactions observed thus far with peptides and amines arinsing from conventional discovery strategies begins to suggest that there may be a limited repertoire of response mechanisms that may be elicitable by many different substances (see Bloom 1984a,b, for fuller discussion). As we and other continue to try to define these response mechanisms, important lessons will undoubtedly be learned for the advancement of our science through the molecular characterization of more substances.

References

Bloom FE (1984a) The functional significance of neurotransmitter diversity. Am J Physiol 246: C184–C194

Bloom FE (1984b) Chemical integrative processes in the central nervous system. In: Handbook of chemical neuroanatomy, vol 2, pp 1–22

Ferron A, Siggins GR, Bloom FE (1984) Vasoactive intestinal polypeptide acts synergistically with noradrenaline to depress spontaneous discharge rates in cerebral cortical neurons. Proc Natl Acad Sci USA 82:8810–8814

Foote SL, Morrison JH (1984) Postnatal development of laminar innervation patterns by mono-aminergic fibers in monkey (*Macaca fascicularis*) primary visual cortex. J Neurosci 4:2667–2680

Foote SL, Bloom FE, Aston-Jones G (1983) Nucleus locus ceruleus: new evidence of anatomical and physiological specificity. Physiol Rev 63:844–914

Magistretti PJ, Morrison JH (1985) VIP neurons in the neocortex. Trends Neurosci 8:7–8

Magistretti PJ, Schorderet M (1985) Norepinephrine and histamine potentiate the increases in cyclic adenosine $3':5'$-monophosphate elicited by vasoactive intestinal polypeptide in mouse cerebral cortical slices: mediation by α_1-adrenergic and H_1-histaminergic receptors. J Neurosci 5:363–368

Morrison JH, Magistretti PJ (1983) Monoamines and peptides in cerebral cortex: contrasting principles of cortical organization. Trends Neurosci 6:146–151

Schmitt FO (1984) Molecular regulators of brain function: a new view. Neuroscience 4:994–1004

Siggins GR, Gruol DL (1986) Synaptic mechanisms in the vertebrate central nervous system. In: Bloom FE (ed) Intrinsic regulatory systems of the brain. Handbook of physiology. The American Physiological Society, Besthesda, Maryland (in press)

Sutcliffe JG, Milner RJ, Shinnick TM, Bloom FE (1983) Identifying the protein products of brain specific genes with antibodies to chemically synthesized peptides. Cell 33:671–682

Sutcliffe JG, Milner RJ, Gottesfeld JM, Reynolds W (1984) Control of neuronal gene expression. Science 225:1308–1315

Estrogen-induced Accumulation of mRNA in Selected Brain Areas

A. MAGGI and I. ZUCCHI[1]

1. Introduction

In mammals, the brain is one of the organs target for the action of estrogens (Maggi and Perez 1983). In fact, these hormones have been described to accumulate in selected brain areas and nuclear receptors capable of specifically recognizing estrogens have been described in the nervous tissue. Furthermore, several studies indicate that these hormones act in selected areas of the Central Nervous System (CNS) to participate in the control of endocrine, motor and affective functions (Maggi and Perez 1983).

Little is known, at the moment, about the mechanisms by which estrogens modulate the nervous activity. In fact, electrophysiological studies have determined that nervous cells exposed to estrogens for a very short time (ms) show an altered excitability. It is unlikely that such a promt effect is achieved by the mechanism which is thought to be adopted by these hormones in peripheric target tissues: binding to cytosolic or nuclear receptors and induction of transcription of specific genes. On the other hand, biochemical investigations indicate that longer exposures to estrogens may determine an increase in the transcription of genes coding for neurotransmitter receptors (Maggi and Perez 1984; Perez and Maggi, submitted).

In order to acquire a better understanding of the action of estrogens in the CNS it should be determined at which extent these hormones may alter the transcriptional activity of nervous tissue and then the specific genes which are under estrogenic regulation in the CNS should be characterized.

In the present report we are describing our initial studies aimed at individuating estrogen-induced mRNA in the brain of rodents.

2. Results

Total RNA was extracted (Glisin et al. 1974) from ovariectomized rats treated with estradiol benzoate (EB 7.5 μg/rat s.c.) 24 h before the investigation. The amount of

1   Milano Molecular Pharmacology Laboratory, Institute of Pharmacology and Pharmacognosy, University of Milano, Piazza Durante 11, 20131 Milano, Italy

Molecular Aspects of Neurobiology
(ed. by Rita Levi Montalcini et al.)
© Springer-Verlag Berlin Heidelberg 1986

Table 1. Accumulation of RNA 24 h after estradiol benzoate administration (7.5 μg/rat s.c.) in selected areas of ovariectomized rat brain

	No. OBS	Total RNA Control (μg RNA/brain nucleus)	Estrogen	(% Increase vs. control)
Olfactory Bulb	5	171 ± 21	186 ± 21	(8.8)
Cerebellum	5	120 ± 8	162 ± 18	(35)
Cortex	8	121 ± 12	143 ± 13	(18)
Hypothalamus	10	69 ± 6	78 ± 5	(13)
Hippocampus	10	102 ± 4	120 ± 9	(18)
Striatum	5	137 ± 3	149 ± 4	(8)

purified RNA was determined by measuring the absorbance at 260 nm and expressed as μg of RNA/mg fresh tissue. The whole dissected nuclei excised from animals subjected to the hormonal treatment did not show any increase in wet weight. As shown in Table 1 a significant increase of total RNA was observed only in the cerebellum (+35%). However, in all the areas examined the amount of RNA measured in the treated animals was slightly higher than in the controls. Since recently it has been reported by Hahn et al. (Chaudari and Hahn 1983; van Ness et al. 1976) that in the brain of adult rodent a large portion of mRNA is not polyadenylated (poly A-) it was of interest to determine whether estrogens could induce preferentially mRNA polyadenylated (poly A+) or poly A-.

We isolated the two classes of mRNA as described (van Ness et al. 1976). Each determination was performed starting from a single animal. As indicated in Table 2, estrogens may affect the accumulation of both classes on mRNA. Per contra the various areas examined responded differentially to the treatment: estrogens induced preferential accumulation of mRNA poly A+ in hippocampus, striatum and cortex and of poly A- in cerebellum and hypothalamus.

The results reported in Table 2 were partially confirmed by in vitro translation of the isolated messages as shown in Table 3. The mRNAs isolated were translated in vitro utilizing a commercial reticulocyte system (N.E.N.). The reaction was carried out

Table 2. Accumulation of mRNA 24 h after estradiol benzoate administration (7.5 μg/rat s.c.) in selected areas of ovariectomized rat brain

	No. OBS	mRNA poly A+ Control (μg RNA/ brain nucleus)	Estrogen	(% Increase vs. control)	mRNA poly A- Control (μg RNA/ brain nucleus)	Estrogen	(% Increase vs. control)
Olfactory Bulb	5	8.5 ± 0.4	9.9 ± 1.2	(16)	9.5 ± 1.3	11.3 ± 1.5	(19)
Cerebellum	5	6.4 ± 1.1	7.4 ± 1.2	(15)	9.6 ± 1.2	12.7 ± 1.1	(32)
Cortex	8	6.5 ± 0.2	9.1 ± 0.4	(40)	7.9 ± 0.3	8.7 ± 0.5	(10)
Hypothalamus	10	4.9 ± 0.1	5.8 ± 0.9	(18)	7.4 ± 1.5	9.9 ± 2.2	(34)
Hippocampus	10	7.7 ± 1.3	13.1 ± 4.2	(70)	9.4 ± 0.9	11.3 ± 0.9	(20)
Striatum	5	6.3 ± 0.2	9.2 ± 0.9	(46)	7.3 ± 1.5	9.0 ± 1.7	(23)

"IN VITRO" TRANSLATION

CORTEX MRNA OF OVX RATS

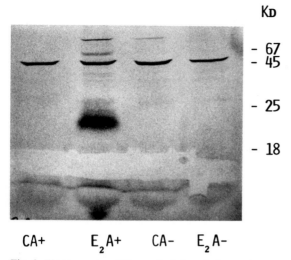

KD

- 67
- 45

- 25

- 18

CA+   E₂A+   CA-   E₂A-

Fig. 1. Fluorography of the analysis by gel electrophoresis of the proteins synthesized in vitro from mRNA isolated from cortex of estrogen-treated (E$_2$ A+, E$_2$ A-) and control (CA+, CA-)-ovariectomized rats. mRNA polyA+ and poly A- are represented by the symbols A+ and A-, respectively. The entire product of the in vitro translation was run on sodium dodecyl sulphate-polyacrylamide gel electrophoresis slab gel (15% total acrylamide) at 33 m A for 4 h. The gel was impregnated with EN³ HANCE (N.E.N.), dried and exposed to Kodak XRP film for 4 days

in presence of 35$_S$ methionine and the quantification of the neosynthesized proteins was performed by trichloroacetic acid precipitation, filtration on Whatman GF/C filters and scintillation counting. In each experiment the nucleic acid translated was the whole amount isolated from the same quantity of starting tissue (in control and treated rats) as determined by weight or DNA content. As predicted on the basis of the observations reported in Table 1, with hypothalamic RNA, the amount of proteins synthesized in presence of mRNA polyA+ was only slightly higher in estrogen primed rats (+13%) while a 30% increase was observed in these animals with mRNA poly A-. Opposite results were observed when mRNA from the cortex was utilized.

The 35$_S$ proteins synthesized utilizing mRNA isolated from the cortex were analyzed by electrophoresis on a gel of 15% polyacrylamide and autoradiography.

Shown in Fig, 1 is the autoradiography were it appears that E$_2$ seems to significantly increase the poly A+ message for a 20 kd protein.

Table 3. In vitro translation of mRNA from cortex and hypothalamus isolated from control and estrogen-treated rats

	Cortex (No. exp.)		Hypothalamus (No. exp.)	
mRNA poly A+ EB / mRNA poly A+ Control	1.36	(3)	1.13	(6)
mRNA poly A- EB / mRNA poly A- Control	0.96	(3)	1.31	(6)

3. Discussion

Our studies indicate that in the rat brain estrogens can influence the accumulation of RNA transcribed by all RNA polymerases, since a significant increase in both total RNA (Table 1) and mRNA (Table 2) was observed.

Interestingly, the extent of the increase in RNAs is not correlated to the distribution of estrogen-receptor (Maggi and Perez 1983). In fact, the hypothalamus, one of the brain areas richest in estrogen-binding activity, does not show the highest accumulation neither of total nor of mRNA. Per contra, a significant increase in mRNA was detected in cortex, an area which does not show estrogen concentrating activity in the adult rat.

It could be postulated that the effect observed in areas (like cortex) poor in estrogen receptors is secundary to the effects elicited by this hormone in the hypothalamus. However, the accumulation of mRNA was observed at a relatively short interval after the hormonal administration (24 h). Furthermore, discrepancies with regard to the presence of steroid hormone receptors and induction of specific steroid-induced product have already been described (De Vellis and Inglish 1968; Leveille et al. 1980). To solve this question we are presently examining the effect of estrogen in vitro on slices of brain tissue. In this system it could also be clarified whether the steroid induced accumulation of RNA is due to neo-synthesis or to inhibition of the catabolism of the nucleic acid.

At the present time the significance of preferential increase on mRNA poly A+ or poly A- in the different areas examined is not understood. Moreover, the quantification of the effect of hormonal administration on mRNA poly A- accumulation is not absolute. In fact, a little percentage of rRNA can be eluted from the benzoylated cellulose at the salt concentration utilized to elute mRNA poly A-.

Therefore, in areas like the cerebellum where estrogens have a strong effect on total RNA accumulation (+35%) it is likely that the poly A- population can be over-extimated. However, in othr areas like the hypothalamus we observed a significant increase in poly A- accumulation (+34%) in spite of the small increase of total RNA (+10%). The data on mRNA poly A- accumulation in hypothalamus were confirmed by in vitro translation of the messages (Table 3). Analysis of one-dimension gel electrophoresis of the products of the in vitro translation of poly A- mRNA did not show any protein product specifically inducible by estrogens. Similar analysis on mRNA poly A+ indicated that in cortex estrogen administration results in an increase of a mRNA coding for a 20K protein which has not been identified yet.

The results presented in this report indicate that one of the mechanisms through which estrogens modulate nervous activity in the brain of mammals is by increasing the accumulation of mRNAs. Certainly, this is only one of the mechanisms adopted by these hormones to influence brain functions since this interaction with the expression of genes cannot be taken into account to explain the rapid alteration of the neuronal firing rate elicited by this steroid (Bueno and Pfaff 1976; Kaba et al. 1983). However, the magnitude of the effect on RNA accumulation suggests that this hormone has a deep influence on the metabolism of cells in the nervous system and encourage to pursue studies aimed at isolating the genes which are specifically induced. Such studies are now feasible with the application of recombinant DNA technologies and are in progress in our laboratory.

Acknowledgments. This work has been supported in part by P.F. Ingegneria Genetica to A.M. and by Hoffmann-La Roche.

References

Bueno J, Pfaff (1976) Single unit recording in hypothalamus and preoptic area of estrogen-treated and untreated overiectomized female rats. Brain Res 101:67–78

Chaudari N, Hahn WE (1983) Genetic expression in the developing brain. Science 220:924–928

De Vellis J, Inglish D (1968) Hormonal control of glycerol phosphate dehydrogenase in rat brain. J Neurochem 15:1061–1070

Glisin V, Crkvenjakov R, Byus C (1974) Ribonucleic acid isolated by cesium chloride centrifugation. Biochemistry 13:2633–2642

Kaba H, Saito H, Otsuka K, Seto K, Kawakami M (1983) Effect of estrogens on the excitability of neurons projecting from the noradrenergic A1 region to the preoptic and anterior hypothalamic area. Brain Res 274:156–159

Leveille PJ, McGinnis JF, Maxwell DS, De Vellis J (1980) Immunocytochemical localization of glycerol phosphate dehydrogenase in rat oligodendrocytes. Brain Res 196:287–305

Maggi A, Perez J (1983) Role of female gonadal hormones in the CNS: clinical and esperimental aspects. Life Scie 37:893–906

Maggi A, Perez J (1984) Progesterone and estrogens in rat brain: modulation of Gaba receptor activity. Eur J Pharmacol 103:165–168

van Ness J, Maxwell IH, Hahn WE (1976) Complex population of non polyadenylated messenger RNA in mouse brain. Cell 18:1341–1349

Perez J, Maggi A (submitted) Estrogen-induced up-regulation of Gaba receptors in the CNS of rodents

Neuronotrophic Activity for CNS Neurons Extracted from Bovine Caudate Nucleus: Partial Purification and Characterization

R. DAL TOSO, O. GIORGI*, D. PRESTI, D. BENVEGNÙ, M. FAVARON,
C. SORANZO, A. LEON, and G. TOFFANO[1]

1. Introduction

The pioneering work of Levi Montalcini and Hamburger (1951) has firmly established the concept that during neuronal ontogeny of the peripheral nervous system (PNS), neuronal survival and neurite outgrowth are regulated by a specific extrinsically occurring neuronotrophic agent termed nerve growth factor (NGF). More recently, it has been proposed that also in the central nervous system (CNS) neuronal survival and neurite number are controlled by extrinsically-occurring neuronotrophic factors (NTF). These agents presumably extend their regulatory activity throughout the whole life span (Varon and Adler 1980; Varon et al. 1983/84) and play an essential role in the restoration of neuronal activity following damage of the adult CNS (Gage et al. 1984).

Whether the isolation of CNS neuronotrophic factors is obtained by means of classical biochemical purification procedures or molecular cloning techniques, their identification is a complex and difficult task since it necessitates assessment of biological activity by means of neuronal cell cultures. To date, although brain extracts or more purified preparations have been reported to enhance neuronal cell survival and neurite outgrowth in vitro, in most cases the effects have been evaluated both by utilizing PNS cultures and by morphological criteria (Barde et al. 1982). CNS cultures have been rarely utilized (Barbin et al. 1984), mainly due to the cell heterogeneity of these cultures.

We here report an investigation directed to detect and purify NTF activity from bovine caudate by analyzing dopaminergic and GABAergic cell development and survival in fetal mouse dissociated mesencephalic cells cultured in serum-free conditions.

1   Fidia Neurobiological Research Laboratories, Via Ponte della Fabbrica 3/A, 35031 Abano Terme, Italy

*   Present address: Istituto Biologico Policattedra, Università di Cagliari, Via Palabanda 12, 09100 Cagliari, Italy

Molecular Aspects of Neurobiology
(ed. by Rita Levi Montalcini et al.)
© Springer-Verlag Berlin Heidelberg 1986

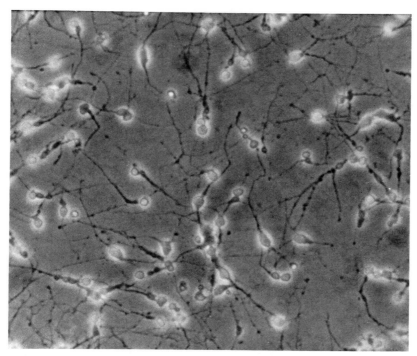

Fig. 1. Phase contrast photomicrograph of fetal mouse dissociated mesencephalic cells at day 4 in vitro. Rostral mesencephalic tegmentum from 13-day mouse embryos was mechanically dissociated, cells centrifuged (45 g × 4 min) and subsequently plated at a density of 1×10^6 cells per 35 mm Falcon tissue culture dishes precoated with bovine skin collagen (Vitrogen, 100 μg protein). The culture medium (2 nm per dish) consisted of a mixture of basal Eagle's medium and Ham's F_{12} (1:1) supplemented with hormone components as described by Di Porzio et al. (1980)

2. Characterization of the Mesencephalic Cell Cultures: Cell Types, Uptake Parameters and Cell Survival

Figure 1 illustrates the typical appearance at phase contrast microscope of dissociated fetal mouse mesencephalic cells cultured for 4 days in a serum-free hormone-supplemented medium. More than 98% of the cells are positively immunoreactive to staining with monoclonal antibody, RT97, known to specifically recognize the 160 kd and 200 kd components of neurofilament protein (Anderton et al. 1982). Quantitative evaluation of dopaminergic cell development and survival was performed by measuring, as a function of time, benztropine (BZT)-sensitive high affinity dopamine (DA) uptake and number of fluorescent neurons (Dal Toso et al., submitted). The DA uptake reached maximal values at day 4 in vitro and subsequently declined. The number of dopaminergic cells remained unvaried up to day 4 (approx. 0.15% of the total seeded cells) and decreased by approximately 75% at day 8 in vitro. DABA-sensitive ^{14}C-GABA uptake and DNA content per plate showed a similar trend. Thus the various neuronal cell types in the culture showed a similar behavior with respect to survival and uptake parameters.

Table 1. Effect of crude supernatant extract or of purified preparations on specific DA and GABA uptake in mesencephalic cell cultures

Addition	BZT-sensitive ^{3}H-DA uptake (fmoles/plate/15 min)	DABA-sensitive ^{14}C-GABA uptake (pmoles/plate/15 min)
Albumin (100 μg)	385 ± 89	8.08 ± 2.00
Supernatant extract (100,000 g × 2 h) 100 μg protein	1026 ± 92	20.21 ± 1.08
Sephadex G-150 (active eluates) 100 μg protein	1056 ± 48	20.51 ± 1.01
HPLC chromatography (active eluate) 2.7 μg protein	1342 ± 96	31.54 ± 0.91
0.27 μg protein	757 ± 111	18.30 ± 2.98
0.027 μg protein	637 ± 20	16.39 ± 0.43

Mesencephalic cells were seeded at a density of 1×10^6 cells/35 dishes in presence of 1.9 ml serum-free medium. After 24 h 100 μl of medium were added containing indicated amounts of protein. When necessary adequate amounts of albumin were also added so as to reach final protein concentration of 100 μg. Specific DA and GABA uptake was evaluated at day 4 in vitro as reported by Prochiantz et al. (1981). Values are mean ± S.E.M. of triplicate analysis. See text for further information

3. NTF Activity in Bovine Caudate Nucleus: Detection and Partial Purification

As observed in Table 1, the addition of dialyzed high speed supernatant fraction (100,000 g × 2 h) of homogenized bovine caudate-nuclei resulted in increase of both BZT-sensitive ^{3}H-DA uptake and DABA-sensitive ^{14}C-GABA uptake when assessed at day 4 in vitro. The effect was dose-dependent (half maximal activity at 10 μg protein) and correlated with an increased survival of the dopaminergic cells and a diminished decline of DNA content per plate at day 8 in vitro. Chemical characterization of the trophic activity indicated that it was heat- (95°C × 30 min) and trypsin-sensitive. When the supernatant extract was applied to a Sephadex G-150 column the trophic activity (Table 1) was eluted approximately in the molecular range of 10–40 kd. Further purification utilizing HPLC cation exchange column chromatography showed that it was solely associated with highly retained molecules active in the ng range. It should be mentioned that the NTF activity is presumably not NGF. In fact addition of NGF to the mesencephalic cultures was totally ineffective in modifying uptake parameters and cell survival. Furthermore, addition of NGF antiserum did not abolish the trophic activity described above.

4. Conclusion and Perspectives

The present results indicate that CNS cultures are valid bioassay systems for detection and quantification of neuronotrophic activity in the brain. Indeed NTF appear to be present in the adult CNS. We are presently trying to purify and characterize the NTF activity and to produce monoclonal antibodies against the NTF. This will permit use of molecular biological techniques and, consequently, analysis of the physiological relevance of the NTF in normal and injured adult mammalian CNS.

References

Anderton BH, Breinburg D, Downes MJ, Green PJ, Tomlinson BE, Ulrich J, Wood JN, Kahn J (1982) Monoclonal antibodies show that neurofibrillary tangles and neurofilaments share antigenic determinants. Nature 298:84–86

Barbin G, Selak I, Manthorpe M, Varon S (1984) Use of central neuronal cultures for detection of neuronotrophic agents. Neuroscience 12:33–43

Barde YA, Edgar D, Thoenen H (1982) Purification of a new neuronotrophic factor from mammalian brain. Embo J 1:549–553

Dal Toso R, Presti D, Benvegnù D, Giorgi O, Vicini S, Azzone GF, Toffano G, Leon A (submitted) Development of phenotypic traits and survival of neurons in dissociated fetal mesencephalic serum-free cell cultures: effects of cell density and stimulation by adult mammalian brain extracts

Di Porzio U, Daguet MC, Glowinski G, Prochiantz A (1980) Effect of striatal cell on in vitro maturation of mesencephalic dopaminergic neurons in serum free conditions. Nature 288:370–373

Gage FM, Björklund A, Stenevi U (1984) Denervation releases a neuronal survival factor in adult rat hippocampus. Nature 308:637–639

Levi Montalcini R, Hamburger V (1951) Selective growth-stimulation effects of mouse sarcoma of the sensory and sympathetic nervous system of the chick embryo. J Exp Zool 116:321–362

Prochiantz A, Daguet MC, Herbert A, Glowinski G (1981) Specific stimulation of in vitro maturation of mesencephalic dopaminergic neurones by striatal membranes. Nature 293:570–572

Varon S, Adler R (1980) Nerve growth factors and control of nerve growth. In: Kevin Hunt R (ed) Current topics in developmental biology, vol 16. Neural development, part II. Neural Development in model systems. Academic Press, New York, p 207

Varon S, Manthorpe M, Williams LR (1983/84) Neuronotrophic and neurite-promoting factors and their clinical potentials. Dev Neurosci 6:73–100

Subject Index